Silence Kills

Medical Humanities

Thomas Mayo, series editor

Silence Kills

Speaking Out and Saving Lives

Edited by

LEE GUTKIND

Foreword by Karen Wolk Feinstein
Introduction by Abraham Verghese

SOUTHERN METHODIST
UNIVERSITY PRESS

Dallas

Requests for permission to reproduce material from this work should be sent to:

Rights and Permissions

Southern Methodist University Press

PO Box 750415

Dallas, Texas 75275-0415

Cover and text design by Tom Dawson

Library of Congress Cataloging-in-Publication Data

Silence kills : speaking out and saving lives / edited by Lee Gutkind ; foreword by Karen Wolk Feinstein ; introduction by Abraham Verghese. — 1st ed.

　　p. cm. — (Medical humanities)

　　ISBN 978-0-87074-518-8 (alk. paper)

　1.　Communication in medicine. 2.　Medical errors.　I. Gutkind, Lee.

　　R118.S55 2007

　　610—dc22

Printed in the United States of America on acid-free paper

10 9 8 7 6 5 4 3 2 1

Contents

Editor's Note

Lee Gutkind

This is *Creative Nonfiction*'s third project devoted to health care. The first, *A View from the Divide*, dealt generally with science, biology, and psychology. It is still in print and has been repeatedly acknowledged by critics and teachers for the fine writing it contains.

Our second collection featured writers who had something significant to say about the need for change in the health care system, especially in the area of patient-professional contact and treatment. The title said it all: *Rage and Reconciliation: Inspiring a Health Care Revolution*. The essays we collected vividly identified the need for change and called for, if not revolution, then a significant and proactive movement to fix a system out of sync with both the people who work within it and those whom it serves.

For *Rage and Reconciliation*, the Jewish Healthcare Foundation (JHF), an organization devoted to supporting health care services, education, and research to encourage medical advancement and protect vulnerable populations, offered a $10,000 prize for the best original narrative essay submitted on the topic. The winner, an attorney and a poet, had been told by a major cancer center that she was dying—that her clock was ticking fast and nothing could be done to help her. She was discouraged from soliciting a second opinion, but she was put off by the arrogance she confronted and, through her persistence, essentially saved herself. Her essay was riveting; her anger palpable. So too was the reaction of our readers—and of our audience at a public forum featuring this writer and one of the angry, frustrated physicians whose work appeared in the collection.

In a review of *Rage and Reconciliation*, the *Journal of the American Medical Association* concluded: "The essays ... are not so much indignant rants as thought-provoking analyses grounded in persuasive evidence that the practical medical problems affecting us all can be rectified only after they have been recognized."

Now we are confronting the health care crisis in an even more vigorous literary assault: *Silence Kills: Speaking Out and Saving Lives*.

Silence Kills, as Jill Drumm's compelling essay explains, was inspired by an initiative of the organizational-performance consulting company Vital Smarts, which in 2005 released a report called *Silence Kills: The Seven Crucial Conversations for Healthcare*. This study soundly concluded that communication breakdown is at the root of most medical errors.

Karen Wolk Feinstein, president of the JHF, and her staff were so impressed with the *Silence Kills* study and so pleased with the circulation and impact of *Rage and Reconciliation* that they approached *Creative Nonfiction* to see if we could bring together writers and health care professionals to address the "silence kills" theme using the vivid storytelling techniques for which creative nonfiction is known. *Silence Kills: Speaking Out and Saving Lives* is the result of this collaboration. Feinstein has provided a foreword to *Silence Kills*, and the introduction is written by Abraham Verghese, the founding director of the Center for Medical Humanities and Ethics at the University of Texas Health Science Center in San Antonio and the author of two powerful memoirs about his experiences as a physician.

A variety of viewpoints are represented in these pages. Three of the contributors to this collection—Paul Austin, Merilee D. Karr, and Helena Studer—are physicians or former physicians, and other essays are written by patients and by patients' and physicians' family members. What their stories have in common is a frustration with a system that hinders communication and, in many cases, leads to unnecessary suffering.

Again, as with *Rage and Reconciliation*, the JHF funded prizes for the best essays. Karr's essay, "Missing," about the experience of being sued for medical malpractice, has been awarded a $1,000 prize for best essay; three runners-up won $500 each: Tamara Dean, for "Saving My Breath"; Pamela Skjolsvik, for "You Have the Right to Remain Silent"; and Grace Talusan, for "Foreign Bodies."

Ordinarily creative nonfiction, as a genre, is inspired by inner feelings and softer (although not necessarily less important) subjects having to do with nature, rural or urban life, or personal survival. Less literary topics are expected to be the province of journalism. We reject this premise as flawed and in many respects elitist; detailed reporting and artful writing are not incompatible. We believe art and literature not only document change but can also inspire and facilitate it. We would not publish any of the essays in *Silence Kills* without believing that our work will fulfill the promise in our subtitle—that speaking out in a dramatic way, with courage and compassion, will save lives and help people to connect and communicate. In choosing the subjects we confront, creative nonfiction writers and editors must listen to our hearts and to our consciences, for the silence of injustice is deafening.

This project involved people from many different organizations, whose contributions to this collection were invaluable. This book would not exist without their help:

- Vital Smarts, especially Marketing & PR Analyst Brittney Maxfield
- Naida Grunden and Nancy Zionts of the Jewish Healthcare Foundation
- Dana Woods of the American Academy of Critical Care Nurses
- Andrew Blauner, our literary agent
- Keith Gregory, Kathryn Lang, and George Ann Ratchford at Southern Methodist University Press
- The staff at *Creative Nonfiction*: managing editor Hattie Fletcher, office manager Julia Ressler, assistant editor Donna Hogarty, and editorial assistant Jess Adamiak

Finally, *Creative Nonfiction* would like to thank the Juliet Lea Hillman Simonds Foundation and the Pennsylvania Council on the Arts for their generous and ongoing support, which makes all our work possible.

Some names and identifying details have been changed to protect the identities of people and institutions mentioned in these essays.

2007

Foreword

Toward a More Caring, and Curing, Health System

Karen Wolk Feinstein

When the Jewish Healthcare Foundation commissioned this project with *Creative Nonfiction*, we had something specific in mind. We wanted to build on a study by the American Association of Critical Care Nurses, also called *Silence Kills*, that highlights how health care professionals avoid conversations crucial to good patient care. Over 50 percent of the 1,700 nurses, doctors, and administrators surveyed have witnessed serious mistakes, broken rules, and incompetence, but only 10 percent ever speak up. Another 25 percent said they'd prefer to leave their jobs or even their professions to avoid confrontations about injurious conditions.

We wanted to use real-life stories to break the code of silence among clinicians about the medical errors and system malfunctions that plague health care. Built into the culture and governance of health care organizations, and exacerbated by overeager and ever-ready malpractice attorneys, is a harmful reticence to disclose, acknowledge, or discuss error. What results is a dangerous, if often inadvertent, collective complicity in harm. If errors aren't disclosed, they can't be fixed. Like Sisyphus pushing his rock uphill, only to have it tumble down again, clinicians are consigned to endless repetition of the same mistakes.

Why? Many fear retaliation for candor and nonconformity. But the results of ignoring serious care problems can be lethal for patients. Hiding behind myriad excuses—It's not my fault; This situation is beyond my control; Bad things happen; I'll lose my job and the trust of my peers—even health care workers with good intentions can be party to behaviors that range from insensitivity to negligence, from unintentional assault to manslaughter.

The Jewish Healthcare Foundation's program-operating arms, the Pittsburgh

Regional Health Initiative and Health Careers Futures, teach a quality-improvement method we call Perfecting Patient Care; its first principle is to treat mistakes and glitches as opportunities for learning, not blame. But, time and again, new trainees face demoralizing resistance from their colleagues. We had hoped to receive essays that would highlight the consequences of this professional "conspiracy," the silent avoidance of problem solving for error reduction.

The essays submitted, however, took us into new waters. We received a host of submissions—not just from health care professionals ruing their silence on medical errors and its aftermath, but from passionate victims (patients and families) of indifferent, careless, and discourteous providers. Certainly, the power of these real tales derives from the underlying emotions—anger, regret, shame, pain—resulting from unsatisfactory care. Beyond the "sin" of silence, healers in these stories reveal a broader host of missteps: disrespect and indifference, incompetence and haste, arrogance, uncertainty, and avoidance. Sometimes what inhibited successful treatment was simply failing to listen, sidestepping complex problems that resist simple solutions, or being overwhelmed by a horror of the real diagnosis. It often turned out to be the patients' or their families' penchant for candid discussions that saved lives and brought healing.

Heroic as many of the patients and their families were in these accounts, they should not have had to resort to extremes to be cared for appropriately, with dignity and respect. It is fashionable, and I would personally prefer, to blame "system" and "organizational" failures and "cultures" for the misadventures in patient care portrayed here and every day in real life. But organizations are collections of individuals, each with their own will and responsibility to protect the people they serve. We need caregivers who confront error and bad judgment, who embrace candor and honesty, the foundations of a new culture of problem solving, risk avoidance, courtesy, and patient centeredness.

There are ways organizations can remove the sense of betrayal among patients, families, and workers. They can adopt a culture of transparency. Dr. Lucian Leape from Harvard Medical School often cites a recent study of several thousand doctors that showed less than half would inform a patient about a serious error and even fewer would provide information to prevent future errors of the same kind.

Instead, Dr. Leape recommends an alternative culture of full disclosure in which health professionals would immediately take responsibility for an error or omission, apologize, and explain what will be done to prevent a recurrence. Evidence suggests patients, families and co-workers respond well to open acknowledgment, sincere apology, and immediate, remedial problem solving. We hope the power of these stories will inspire health care professionals to break rank and cross the barrier of silence.

Karen Wolk Feinstein is president and CEO of the Jewish Healthcare Foundation and chair of the Pittsburgh Regional Healthcare Initiative.

Introduction

Abraham Verghese

The stories in *Silence Kills* might appear to be about medicine. My sense when I was done reading them was that they were really about life, about the very human urge to extend life and relieve suffering, and about how easily in trying to make things better we can make things worse.

I have practiced medicine just long enough to see nearly every trend of the previous decade contradicted in the next one. It is humbling to look back at what we once espoused, and yet our pronouncements of today are just as dogmatic as when we thought lobotomy was the cure for schizophrenia (it isn't), that triglycerides don't matter (they do), or that peptic ulcers can't be infectious (many are caused by *Helicobacter pylori*). I came of age in medicine in the 1980s, which I think of as the grand age of cure; those of us in training were caught up in the conceit of cure. It seemed there was little that we could not tackle or wrestle down with modern medicine, and when we failed we were never to blame. Blame the poor condition of the patient's protoplasm, or the fact the patient came too late. We had chemotherapy to kill off any cancer; it was unfortunate the patient could not withstand the dose. Out of that conceit, I specialized in infectious diseases, which seemed to me to be the one subspecialty in medicine that was all about cure: make an astute diagnosis, and a traveler returned from the Congo with a bizarre rash rises like Lazarus. What could be more rewarding?

Then came our lesson in humility, and it was called HIV. My generation of infectious disease physicians, caught up in the conceit of cure, was now dealing with a fatal disease for which we had nothing to offer, certainly no cure. We found out, almost by accident, that even when we had no cure to offer, if we were willing to leave our medical-industrial complexes, if we were willing to visit patients in their homes, get to know their families, we were paradoxically bringing about a kind of *healing* in the absence of a cure. By healing, I mean that all of us—patient, family, and physician—came to terms with the disease and with mortality, not just that of the patient, but our own. It was the kind of communication and connection with patient and family, the kind of focus on the individual (as opposed to the disease in the individual) that allowed the horse-and-buggy doctor of many years ago to be such a powerful and respected figure; it was the kind of communication that in a technological age we had lost sight of, or thought was not important.

The ascendance of technology in the last two decades is mind-boggling. I have stood with radiologists in front of their banks of monitors and watched them "reconstruct" a three-dimensional view of a liver before my eyes in order to see a spot that concerns me. Then, with a click of the mouse, the radiologist shows me the blood supply to the liver—arteries in vivid red—even turning the liver this way and that as if it were a piece of clay mounted on a wheel. The striking thing is that my presence in the same room as the radiologist has become unusual. In our wired world, I can pull up the X-ray image (albeit a simpler version) and the radiologist's report at my desk, or even at home. Yet, it was all those times we traipsed down to Radiology after rounds to look at our patients' films, all those times that we lassoed a passing radiologist to give us an opinion, to ask questions, to learn, to be educated, that have left me with some skill in looking at such images. How sad that the next generation will not get that kind of informal learning, and may not get to form a personal relationship with a colleague in radiology. My radiologist friends, who might have grudged the disruption of our visits, now bemoan the fact that they rarely see us. They miss hearing the stories of the people whose shadows they study; they have to be content with the cryptic "chest X-ray, rule out pneumonia" on our electronic requisition. From a "systems" point of view this is most efficient; from a clinician's viewpoint and from the point of view of a hospital's esprit de corps, which is built on relationships, it is a loss.

• • •

A parallel phenomenon is the near extinction of "bedside rounds," that hallowed tradition of teaching hospitals. Rounds are now too often conducted in a conference room with nary a patient to be seen. I have come under fire for saying that I think the patient in the bed has become a mere icon for the *real* patient who is in the computer. But it is true. Interns and residents quickly find that the ebb and flow of a patient's short hospital stay (so short it borders on illogical) revolves around getting tests requested, getting results back, requesting consults, getting the opinions back, and scheduling procedures. The workspace for this activity is not the nurses' station and the chart rack (once a great place to meet and discuss patients with nurses and other physicians), and it's not the bedside of the patient. The "work" takes place in the electronic medical record accessed from the "desktop" of a computer in a nook somewhere. The echocardiograms and CT scans and endoscopy images of the patient's innards, the numbers that describe the blood and organ functions, and ergo, the real patient, is *in* the computer, visible to you with password and screen. The breathing, talking, anxious person in the bed, who wonders why the doctors appear so busy and yet so rarely come by, is an abstract entity.

Patients grudgingly admire and seek the incredible things medicine has to offer— indeed, they are conditioned to expect miracles—but they are wary because there is a price to pay (and let's not talk about monetary costs here). The price of cutting-edge technology is the sense you have that your medical care feels impersonal, distant, with no one person truly in control. Your doctor, who has cared for you for years, admits you to a *hospitalist* when you need to be admitted. (Hospitalists are in-house and familiar with hospital systems and with acute, in-hospital care, and so this is not a bad trend—better, one could argue, than having your doctor whip by for a few minutes at the start or the tail end of a busy office day. Even if it is better, however, the fact is that you miss your doctor's familiar face, you miss the person who is supposed to know the most about your body.) Medical care has become so specialized, you are very likely to see many other new faces, new specialists in the hospital. You might feel you are being pieced out: your heart to the *non-invasive* cardiologist, who might call in the *invasive* cardiologist if you need a cardiac catheterization, who, if you need angioplasty or a stent, gets the *interventional* cardiologist, who, if the root problem is a bad heart rhythm, calls in the cardiac *electrophysiologist.*

So much can go wrong even in the best hands when such complex care is being delivered. When the Institute of Medicine, under Dr. Kenneth Shine's visionary leadership, released its 1999 report *To Err Is Human: Building A Safer Health System*, we physicians were more surprised than the public. We were aware of our screwups, but in our conceit we assumed (or we hoped) that overall they were minor in comparison to the good we did, the lives we saved. The now-infamous statistic in the IOM report was that the number of people who die from medical errors each day was the equivalent of a jumbo jet full of people crashing. It is an unforgettable metaphor, but it both understates and overstates the problem. It does not cover the little instances of neglect, minor for the system but huge for the patient and family—for example, a patient kept without food for an early morning procedure who finds out only in the late afternoon that the procedure is postponed to the next day. The jumbo jet metaphor overstates the problem in that it presupposes that medicine is delivered by something other than fallible humans. In addition, sometimes we waste billions on futile but expensive care in the last days of a life, because we are unable as a society to ration resources and unwilling to call it quits. At one level, then, we make more medical mistakes because we simply do more medically than we should, and we do it to people who have little chance of recovery and a good chance of getting worse from our efforts.

Much has changed in the light of the Institute of Medicine report. The electronic medical record saves lives and saves us from many mistakes, but it also means your doctor is half-turned away from you at your visit, busy typing, and so misses the consternation on your face, misses your body language of annoyance, because the courtesies you expect even of your third grader ("Look at me when I talk to you") are not in evidence.

Though I am board-certified in two subspecialties in internal medicine, increasingly I see my role for my patients in this era of complex care as that of a new kind of specialist: the quarterback. Often I admit patients even though their problem is not in my discipline, because it is the quickest way to expedite the handoff to a star specialist or to get them a procedure they need. I must daily survey the field and weigh the evolving knowledge of what ails the patient against my personal knowledge of the professional expertise in my community; I must huddle with the family and interpret and weave a complete story out of the little fragments and snippets they receive from the myriad of professionals who come and go from the room; I must call the next play and give my reasons. The consultants up in the booth give me their recommendations, often grounded in science, in "evidence-based" medicine; I must weigh that against the other evidence I smell and see on the ground, evidence that revolves around such ephemeral things as a quaver in the voice, an expression in the face of someone I have come to know over many visits, a knowledge of the toll of this hospitalization on the pocketbook, on the family future; I take old-fashioned soundings such as the state of the pulse, the coating of the tongue, the cogency of thoughts and words, the turgor of the skin, the feel of the belly, the nature of tendon reflexes and the gait. I am often wrong by the measures of science, and I risk the wrath of the consultant who will be justifiably annoyed that I am second-guessing in an area that is not my area of expertise; but wrong or right, I am responsible. There are times to go for broke, the Hail Mary pass. There are times to concede that there is no cure, and to work on the healing; there are times to take a knee and settle for what we have rather than go for perfection; often it is a draw, and we hope we can regroup and prevail in overtime.

Reading these essays—the experiences they recount, the painful realizations and the illness, suffering, and frustrations they describe—is to hear a cry for a return to a simpler, more personal kind of medical care. *Talk to me!* These essays strive to break the silence, to ask the questions that should be asked, that should have been asked. They illustrate how easily pride, misunderstanding, laziness, denial, poor data-gathering, avarice, expediency, selfishness and, above all, poor communication can undo the best of technology, the best that medicine has to offer.

Sometimes I think we in medicine are guilty of thinking that medicine is now all science, and that the "art" was just for the old days. Sometimes I think we inadvertently convey this message to our students. But this collection proves otherwise; the practice of medicine today needs science *and* art, each in equal measure. The "art" in medicine lies in our willingness to recognize that it is an art. The art requires well-trained people to listen, hear, think, and walk in the shoes of the patient, if for no other reason than that one day we will all walk in those shoes.

Abraham Verghese is the director of the Center for Medical Humanities
and Ethics at the University of Texas Health Science Center, San Antonio, where he holds
the Joaquin Cigarroa Jr. Chair and the Marvin Forland Distinguished Professorship.
He is the author of *My Own Country* and *The Tennis Partner*.

The Good Doctor

Helena Studer

Stop.

What?

I said, stop.

Why?

Because you're in the wrong lung.

No, I'm not.

You're in the wrong lung. Just look at the fluoro.

Oh, my God.

Have you taken biopsies?

Yes.

Just stop.

Twenty minutes before Dr. John Riley stepped back into the bronchoscopy suite of University Hospital and uttered the word "stop," the day seemed promising. As an attending physician at one of the largest lung transplant centers in the country, Riley enjoyed being on the Bronchoscopy Service. His day was filled with bronchoscopies—procedures that involve technical prowess and precision. Performing procedures gave him immediate satisfaction and results, and he was good at them.

John Riley's decision to work with a dying population of patients, as most lung transplants are, seems incongruous when one first meets this affable, almost lighthearted man. Inclined to humor, liked by his colleagues and patients, Riley fosters a sense that he is easygoing. He nicknamed one patient "Santa" because of the patient's uncanny resemblance to the mythological character, and actually addresses the patient as "Santa"—much to the chagrin of his colleagues and the unending amusement of his patient. But he approaches his work and his patients in a measured, meticulous fashion. His colleagues describe him as an excellent doctor and have seen him rounding at the hospital until ten o'clock at night, attending to his patients. John Riley uses the absurd as a shield because he treats emotionally demanding patients like lung transplants: patients who routinely require ten to twelve medications each, are frequently hospitalized in intensive care units because they are immune-suppressed, and undergo at least six bronchoscopies just in the first year after transplantation.

A lung transplant is a treatment of last resort. After a patient undergoes lung transplantation for a chronic lung disease like emphysema or cystic fibrosis, bronchoscopies become part of a vigilant plan to detect infection or rejection of the donor/transplanted lung. Infection and, eventually, rejection frequently cause death in lung transplant patients. According to the most recent data collected by the United Network for Organ Sharing (UNOS), survival after lung transplantation is only 47 percent nationally at five years.

In order to monitor for the two most common causes of death in transplant patients—infection and rejection—doctors need to look directly at the transplanted lung and take a biopsy, a piece of the lung. A bronchoscopy accomplishes that goal. Unfortunately, it is invasive—it necessitates physically entering and manipulating the body. It falls under the category of same-day surgery, with risks of bleeding, infection, puncture of the lung (pneumothorax), and even death.

University Hospital's lung transplant team prides itself on a survival rate well above the national average, despite the fact that it performs lung transplants on higher-risk patients than most other centers in the country. The team cites the cumulative experience its members and the hospital staff gain from the sheer volume of lung transplants they perform each year, working in one of the largest centers in the country. In other words, the more transplants they do, the more experience they gain, and the better they get. Their claim is supported by several studies published in two of the most prominent journals in medicine, the *New England Journal of Medicine* and the *Journal of the American Medical Association*, which agree that high-volume centers have better outcomes. University Hospital's morbidity rate—the number of patients who suffer side effects after a bronchoscopy—is also lower than the national average.

• • •

When Thelma Jones appeared on a stretcher before the large steel double doors leading to the bronchoscopy suite, she was greeted as usual by Paul, the lead nurse. I imagine their conversation went like this:

"It's you again, Thelma? Is it that time already?"

Thelma tried to laugh. "Actually, Paul, I don't feel too good this time."

"I'm sorry to hear that, Thelma. Are you having trouble breathing and coughing more than normal?"

"Yes."

"I guess that means it's not a surveillance bronch. We're looking for something. Well, you've been here so much you know the routine, right?"

"Yes."

"I still need you to sign the consent for the bronch that the docs are gonna do."

"I know."

"Is your son gonna wait for you?"

"Yes."

"Now remind me, Thelma, which lung did we transplant in you?"

"The left one."

Chatting about Thelma's house in the remote Upper Peninsula of Michigan, her son driving her the many hours into the city, and the lack of parking around the hospital, Paul wheeled Thelma into the white-tiled procedure room. As he hooked up the heart monitor to her chest and the pulse oximeter to her right index finger, Frank, the bronch technician, prepared for the bronchoscopy. Already suited up in his blue lead-filled apron to protect against the radiation used during the procedure, Frank was also masked, gowned, and gloved. Carefully he laid out the instruments on a metal tray: tiny metal forceps, syringes filled with sterile saline and 1 percent lidocaine, plastic tubes and containers for specimens to be collected, and the black bronchoscope with its bulky camera lens and portals at one end followed by a long, narrow cylindrical tail containing flexible fiber-optic bundles. Images from that camera would be transmitted to a seventeen-inch television monitor bolted to the ceiling above the patient. All those involved with the procedure could see where in the lung the bronchoscope was located.

The camera of the bronchoscope would be blinded by mucous and blood at the moment the metal forceps took biopsies, however, and so fluoroscopy or X-ray capability was also necessary so that the doctors could see where they were in the lung. A radiopaque image, tracing the bronchoscope from the vocal cords, past the trachea, down the bronchi and bronchioles into lung parenchyma, would show where the metal forceps grabbed a piece of lung. These X-ray images would be projected onto circular screens below the rectangular bronchoscope screen. The color images on the bronchoscope screen would move; the images on the fluoro screen would be freeze-frames in black and white.

Frank would turn on the fluoroscopy engine last, because the din of that machine would compete with any other sound in the room, including the rhythmic beeps from the monitors sounding out Thelma Jones's heart.

While preparations were going on, Bill White, a physician in training, stepped into the room to speak with Thelma Jones. A tall, broad-shouldered man, Bill inspired confidence in the people he worked with. All those involved in this case describe a competent physician, someone with adequate knowledge, a trainee with several years of experience. He was not a greenhorn, nor was he disparaged by the bronchoscopy staff as a "box-of-rocks."

By all accounts, Bill White introduced himself and reviewed with Thelma Jones the details of the bronchoscopy: she would be sedated, numbing medicine would be applied to her vocal cords, the bronchoscope inserted, and washings and biopsies taken. Bill also discussed with Thelma Jones the possible side effects of a bronchoscopy—excessive bleeding or a punctured lung being the most common. But he assured her that at University Hospital, the incidence of either happening was less than 1 percent, significantly lower than the 2–3 percent reported nationally. What he didn't tell her was what would happen if the wrong lung was biopsied.

"The patient is on the table" are the words the bronch staff uses to tell an attending physician, like John Riley, that his presence is required for a bronch. Riley does not remember those words being spoken that day, however. He remembers briefly speaking with Thelma Jones in the bronch suite. He recalls meeting with the nurse manager of the bronch suite in her office, then walking down the hall with her to the procedure room. He thinks he partially propped the door open as they finished their conversation about patient safety. Then he stepped into the procedure room and into what he later described as the worst nightmare of his professional life.

Riley's eyes flicked to the fluoro screen and froze. He saw the image of the bronchoscope in the black and white shadows of Thelma's right lung.

"What is going on here?" he asked with disbelief in his voice.

Bill turned his face, shielded behind an orange mask and plastic eye guard.

"We're doing the bronch."

But Bill knew that as a trainee he was not supposed to go past the vocal cords without an attending physician in the bronch room.

"Where do you think you are?"

"In the left lung."

"Stop." John Riley tried to control the panic in his voice.

"What?"

"I said, *stop.*"

"Why?"

"Because you're in the wrong lung."

"No, I'm not."

Before John Riley could respond, Frank, the bronch tech, chimed in. "What are you talking about, John? Bill's in the right lung."

"That's my point. He's in the *right* lung, not the left. We transplanted Thelma's left lung," John Riley answered.

"I'm in the left lung." Bill defended his position. Paul, who had his back toward the procedure while he was charting Thelma Jones's vital signs, turned and looked at the fluoro screen.

"The hell you are," he said flatly.

"I did not go into the wrong lung. I'm telling you, I'm in the left lung," Bill persisted.

"You're in the wrong lung. I'm sure of it. Just look at the fluoro."

As John Riley uttered those words, Bill glanced upward. His gaze locked on the fluoro screen. There was no denying it; the silhouette of Thelma Jones's heart, the shadows of her ribs, clearly showed he had gone into her right lung, her nontransplanted lung. The wrong lung.

"Oh, my God."

"Have you taken biopsies?" John Riley asked tensely.

"Yes." A single word that spoke volumes.

Bill had overstepped his bounds by proceeding past the vocal cords without an attending surgeon in the bronchoscopy room. But taking biopsies without an attending surgeon flagrantly disregarded the policy of physician-trainee behavior.

"Just stop. Just stop and pull out the scope."

The ensuing silence seemed to press on John Riley's shoulders. He slumped as he crossed his arms and fixated on the image of Thelma Jones's right lung on the fluoro screen. The image would remain frozen there until a new picture was snapped. He scanned for evidence of a pneumothorax, or air trapped between the lung and the chest wall. A pneumothorax during a bronchoscopy is a dangerous consequence of puncturing the lung and air leaking from the lung into the pleural space. The pleural space is hemmed in by the bony sternum, ribcage, and spine. As air fills the pleural space, it pushes against the lung until it causes the lung to collapse.

To illustrate the result of a pneumothorax, John Riley describes a scene from the movie *Dances with Wolves*: an arrow is shot into a herd of bison thundering across the American Plains. The arrow pierces the right chest wall of a large male bison, shattering bone, tearing muscle, causing air to rush into the pleural cavity. The bison labors to keep running. But he can't breathe; air has collected in a space where it doesn't belong, squeezing both his lungs until they shrivel like deflated balloons. Oxygen no longer flows to his heart, his kidneys, his brain. Soon he crashes to the ground, a dead brown heap.

But bison have only one pleural space, while humans have two distinct pleural spaces, one surrounding each lung. In Thelma Jones's case, a pneumothorax causing collapse or "dropping" her right lung would not be imminently life-threatening if she could still breathe with her left lung. But the reason she was in the bronch suite in the first place was because they needed to biopsy her left lung, her transplanted lung, the lung that Riley suspected Thelma Jones was rejecting.

Performing a biopsy on a lung always runs the risk of a pneumothorax. Obtaining a biopsy of Thelma Jones's right lung had been useless. Worse, it may have placed her life in peril. The woman was sick. If she was rejecting her transplanted lung, only a biopsy of her left lung could give them the answer. John Riley was caught between the proverbial rock and a hard place. If he did not biopsy her left lung now and she was rejecting, then he was delaying diagnosis and life-saving treatment. If he biopsied her left lung now and she "dropped" both her lungs, she could die. An opportunity wasted or a risk of death.

As the attending physician, John Riley had to make the decision. Ultimately he was responsible. He decided to get a higher resolution X-ray than the fluoro could provide. Because air rises, a pneumothorax of the right upper lobe of the lung should show up more clearly if they sat the patient upright and took an X-ray. If there was no evidence of a pneumo on the right side, they could bronch her left lung as intended, although they still ran the risk of giving her a pneumo on the left side.

While they waited for a radiologist to give them an official reading, Riley pulled Bill aside.

"What happened back there?"

Implicit in the question was John Riley's anger.

"I'm sorry."

"Bill, you went into the wrong lung."

"I'm sorry."

"How did that happen?"

"I don't know. Look, John, I'm really sorry."

"We'll get through this. We just have to deal with what happened."

Those were the only words John Riley said in response to Bill's attempt to seek reassurance. Bill probably wanted Riley to say that it was OK; he wanted someone to forgive him for making a mistake. But it was not OK. A patient had suffered consequences, and everyone in that room had played a part.

When the reading of the X-ray came back as "no pneumo," the relief was palpable on Riley's face. But it was cold comfort. He knew that they had transplanted Thelma Jones because of emphysema, and emphysematous lungs are more likely to develop a pneumothorax after biopsy because of their friable nature. So the fact that Thelma Jones's right lung, her emphysematous lung, was biopsied and showed no evidence of a pneumothorax remained unsettling.

They combed every inch of the right lung with the fluoroscope. Still no evidence of a pneumothorax.

They bronched Thelma Jones's left lung, taking washings and biopsies quickly and efficiently. They scanned her left lung for evidence of a pneumo and found none. Then they scanned her right lung again. This time, a pneumothorax was plainly visible in the right upper lobe. As Riley had feared, mistakenly biopsying her emphysematous lung had resulted in a pneumo.

"I'm sorry" were the only words spoken. Bill's remorse permeated the silence.

All they could do was wait and see if a pneumothorax would also develop in Thelma Jones's left lung. If she had pneumothoraxes of both her lungs, she could become that bison in *Dances with Wolves*.

The treatment for a pneumothorax entails inserting a chest tube between the ribs and sucking out the pocket of air in the pleural space, allowing the lungs to reexpand and the patient to breathe. Thelma Jones was fortunately still under anesthesia when a clear, plastic catheter was emergently pierced into her right chest wall between the third and fourth ribs. But because she was still under anesthesia, she could not be informed about the consequences of her bronchoscopies. Riley had to inform her next of kin, her son.

"We need to speak about what happened during your mother's procedure today." Riley started the conversation as soon as they sat down in the bronchoscopy suite conference room.

"Is something wrong, Dr. Riley?"

"I need to inform you that a complication occurred during your mother's procedure."

"What happened?"

"While there are times that we biopsy the native lung as well as the transplanted lung in order to get better answers, that was not the case with your mother today. We only intended to biopsy her left lung, her transplanted lung. Inadvertently, we biopsied your mother's right lung."

Riley paused. "As a result of that biopsy, your mother developed a pneumo-thorax. We punctured her lung; it should not have happened."

"Are you saying you made a mistake?"

"Sometimes when we are in the lungs, the bronchoscope becomes obscured by mucous or blood and we get turned around. In your mother's case, we went into the right lung instead of the left lung and took a biopsy where we should not have. It was not our intention. It should not have happened."

Thelma Jones's son must have heard the distress in John Riley's voice, must have read the anguish on his face.

"I understand that mistakes happen. I understand that sometimes, even in the best of circumstances, things go wrong. My mother and I appreciate the care you have always given her. She wouldn't be here without you taking care of her. I know you did your best."

Thelma Jones's son sounded almost consoling.

John Riley has never been named as a defendant in a medical malpractice suit. And he wants to keep it that way. He knows that half of all physicians, regardless of ability or error, are sued during the course of their careers. As calculated as it may sound, Riley was very careful not to say the word "sorry." Hospital risk-management lawyers have advised him that in the current medical-legal environment, that word is tantamount to an admission of fault and therefore an invitation to be sued. Some patients and their families hear "sorry" and immediately assign blame and take punitive action. Of medical malpractice claims, 40 percent are without merit, according to a study published in the May 2006 *New England Journal of Medicine.*

But John Riley wanted to say that he was sorry. It weighs on his conscience that Thelma Jones's son, and Thelma herself, when she was informed, were both so understanding about his part in a serious medical error. Riley does not deny that a mistake occurred; he readily admits he was ultimately responsible. Nor does he blame his trainee; he says he failed his patient in adequately assuring her safety and he failed his trainee in adequate supervision. He lives with his failure—his failure of human error.

The Institute of Medicine (IOM) in its 1999 report *To Err Is Human: Build-*

ing A Safer Health System claims that as many as 44,000 to 98,000 people die in hospitals each year as the result of medical errors. This makes medical errors the eighth leading cause of death in the United States—ahead of car accidents, breast cancer, and AIDS. Two weeks after the IOM released its report, the Clinton administration issued an executive order instructing government agencies to implement techniques for reducing medical errors, and Congress launched a series of hearings on patient safety. Yet medical errors continue to plague the nation. Four years after the IOM report was issued, one expert in medical error declared that he could not "find evidence that health care in the United States is becoming safer."

The Institute of Medicine defines medical error as "the failure of a planned action to be completed as intended or the use of a wrong plan to achieve an aim." Most medical errors are preventable. According to one landmark study on medical error, over 75 percent of adverse events were either preventable or potentially preventable. What the IOM calls an "epidemic" of medical errors costs the nation an estimated $17 billion to $29 billion each year, with no end in sight. Beyond the cost in human lives and dollars, however, is the unquantifiable cost in the "loss of trust" by patients and the "loss of morale and frustration" by doctors.

What surprised many people, but should not have, is one of the IOM report's main conclusions: "The majority of medical errors do not result from individual recklessness or the actions of a particular group—this is not a 'bad apple' problem. Most commonly, errors are caused by faulty systems, processes, and conditions that lead people to make mistakes or fail to prevent them." In other words, medical error is not about one bad doctor or even a group of them; it is about the controllable conditions or situations under which even a good doctor makes a mistake. The IOM report clearly states that "mistakes can best be prevented by designing the health system at all levels to make it safer—to make it harder for people to do something wrong and easier for them to do it right." This means changing the "error-prone" environment in which doctors practice medicine. It means correcting what Lucian Leape, a leading expert in medical error, calls "defects in the design" of systems that lead good doctors to make mistakes that are often "no different from the simple mistakes people make everyday." In his article "Institute of Medicine Medical Error Figures Are Not Exaggerated," published in the *Journal of the American Medical Association*, Leape agrees with the IOM that medical errors result from faulty systems, not faulty people. Furthermore, he contends that "errors are excusable; ignoring them is not."

The IOM report also argues that "blaming an individual does little to make the system safer and prevent someone else from committing the same error." Yet, according to a study published in 2002 by the *New England Journal of Medicine*, "Views of Practicing Physicians and the Public on Medical Errors," the public remains unwilling to accept this. When asked what they considered one of the most important problems with health care and medicine, much of the public responded with the term "incompetent doctors." Half of respondents viewed the suspension of licenses of doctors as an effective way to reduce medical errors. The public believes that doctors, not systems or processes, are primarily responsible for medical errors and should be sued, fined, and subject to suspension of their professional licenses. They cling to the notion that only bad doctors are responsible for bad mistakes. The American public doesn't want to hear that good doctors make mistakes and perfection in medicine is impossible.

What does not weigh on John Riley's conscience is silence. As tempting as it was to tell Thelma Jones and her son that a biopsy was planned of her right lung and that the pneumothorax was the unfortunate outcome of a necessary procedure, John Riley chose to tell the truth. I admire him for that. I know just how easy it is to be silent. Many years ago, I witnessed an ob-gyn make a terrible mistake during a routine hysterectomy. I stood in the operating room retracting the patient's belly open while he carelessly hacked out her ovary. I stood next to her hospital bed as he lied to her about his mistake.

"We had to take the right ovary, Gina."

"Why? What happened?"

"Jesus Christ, Gina. It was a mess in there."

"I'm sorry."

She apologized. As if it was her fault that he had butchered her ovary.

He offered no other explanations. Yet I did not speak up when this incident occurred. I was a medical student with my career in front of me; he was an attending surgeon. I participated in the complicity of silence.

John Riley's honesty earned him a meeting with the hospital administration and the director of clinical operations for a *root cause analysis*—a meeting John Riley describes as one in which everyone else was dressed, but he had "no pants on." And he repeatedly had to admit to the mistake for over an hour.

The hospital administrator stared at him over her half-moon glasses.

"Dr. Riley, were you present at the beginning of the procedure?"

"No, I was not."

"Why?"

"I was distracted by my administrative duties. But I know that I should have been there."

"Why did no one else in the room pick up the error?"

"It was not their job. It was mine."

"But you don't deny that the lead nurse or the bronchoscopy technician had the experience to detect the error."

"I don't deny that. The lead nurse was instrumental in confirming that the trainee had biopsied the wrong lung. But the fact remains that it was not anyone else's job but mine to monitor the trainee."

"Dr. Riley, why did the trainee make the error?"

"I don't know. I can only surmise that he became disoriented and biopsied the wrong lung."

"Was there anything you could have done to prevent the error?"

"Yes. I should have been there. I could have stopped him from biopsying the wrong lung."

"Dr. Riley, did the patient have an adverse event due to the error?"

"Yes, the patient suffered significant morbidity."

"What happened to the patient?"

"She had a pneumothorax. She required a chest tube as well as an admission to the intensive care unit."

"Dr. Riley, are admissions to the intensive care unit routine after a bronchoscopy?"

"No. It was a result of our error."

As a physician myself, I imagined John Riley's experience in that *root cause analysis* like a deposition in a medical malpractice suit, though he maintains that the interrogation probably did not go as harshly as I envisioned it. Nonetheless, he acknowledges that it was painful and uncomfortable. He remembers many times wanting to get up and leave. But he does not wish he had kept silent. Because, as predicted by the Institute of Medicine, when mechanisms exist for the examination of a medical error, specific things can be learned and similar errors of process can be prevented.

Productive changes resulted from John Riley's humiliation. At University Hospital, a radiopaque "YES" now marks the side of the chest where a bronchoscopy is to be done. Everyone in the bronchoscopy suite, from the attending to the bronch tech, checks for the "YES" before proceeding to a biopsy. Also, the bronch staff routinely conducts a "time-out"—for example, the physician performing the bronchoscopy might say, "It is Tuesday morning. The time is 10:15 and we are doing a bronch of Mr. Smith's right lung. Does everyone agree?" A chorus of agreement must be heard from every member of the bronch team or the procedure is stopped. And no one allows a trainee to go past the vocal cords without an attending present. Now, before John Riley does any bronch, every single time he will say something like this: "Mr. Smith, we did a transplant of your right lung. Is that right? OK, then, today we are going to do a bronchoscopy of your right lung."

But how many doctors are willing to subject themselves to a detailed examination of their error? The answer seems to be: not many. In the *New England Journal of Medicine* study "Views of Practicing Physicians and the Public on Medical Errors," only one-fifth of physicians thought that voluntary reporting of serious medical errors to a state agency would be very effective in preventing them. Equally disturbing is what one expert called the "relative blindness" of physicians to the high frequency and relative severity of medical errors. Although nearly one-third of physicians reported witnessing an error and over half of those believed that a similar error was very likely to recur, most physicians still believe that individual doctors are to blame for preventable medical errors. Physicians remain resistant to the idea espoused by the Institute of Medicine that errors are primarily failures of institutional systems rather than failures of individuals. Doctors, like their patients, seem wedded to the notion that perfection is possible in medicine.

Thelma Jones did not develop a pneumothorax of her left lung. The pneumothorax of her right lung resolved with treatment, and she was transferred from the ICU to a regular floor within forty-eight hours and then discharged. Unfortunately, she rejected her transplanted left lung. She died six months after this incident. Whether this incident contributed to her death is questionable; chronic rejection eventually results in death, no matter the treatment.

I asked John Riley how often the wrong lung is biopsied during a bronchoscopy.

"I don't know," he answered. "We don't keep track of our mistakes."

Helena Studer, a former assistant professor of pediatrics, no longer practices pediatrics. She is currently at work on a collection of essays examining the tension between the technology of medicine and the human factor.

Missing

Merilee D. Karr

I stared down at my name neatly typed next to the word "Defendant." Around it were numbers, names, and small print that I didn't understand, on a form headlined "In the Circuit Court of the State of Oregon."

Below my name, small print said, "You are hereby required to appear and defend the complaint filed against you—" What complaint? More neat typing filled another blank line: "the Estate of Helen F. Simmons, Deceased." Helen? I knew her. Curly brown hair, funny lady. Deceased? Oh, no. She was only in her forties, but she'd already had at least one heart attack. I realized I hadn't seen her for a while. Deceased? My god, what had happened?

The next page was a different legal form, with numbers down the left edge. This, too, repeated the heading "In the Circuit Court of the State of Oregon." Just below the heading, in capital letters, was, "ESTATE OF HELEN F. SIMMONS, DECEASED, PLAINTIFF, VS. MERILEE D. KARR, M.D., DEFENDANT." And next to that was the answer I was looking for: "Complaint: Wrongful Death Based on Medical Negligence."

Oh, my god. Deceased. It was me. I killed her. My knees buckled, I couldn't breathe, and I wanted to dig a hole in the floor and disappear into it.

That form was a supoena. That's how I heard about my first malpractice suit.

Finally. It was like I'd been waiting for this. I had finally screwed up. For real. Through medical school, residency training, and my own medical practice, up to that day and since—with every decision I've ever made in any patient's care—I've grilled myself: *What if this is wrong? Isn't there a better way to do this? What else might this person have that I haven't heard of or thought of? What if I'm wrong?*

We all do it, on this end of the stethoscope. And now a woman was dead, and I was no longer the only one accusing me of negligence and malpractice. All the doubt that came with my diploma slammed home. Finally I knew. I just wasn't good enough.

As I stood staring at the subpoena, the bustle and chatter of a workday swirled around me, and I suddenly realized that the whole clinic knew. The nurses, billing clerks, and lab techs detoured around my desk. I was in everyone's path—the doctors shared a row of desks in a central work area. No one had spoken to me since the subpoena had captured my eye—under other circumstances I would have enjoyed such a long stretch of uninterrupted time. Even the other doctors hadn't interrupted my ruminations. I wondered what they were thinking. I didn't look up to see if anybody was staring at me. Didn't want to embarrass anyone.

I was the new doctor in this group—I had joined fresh out of residency two years before—and now I had brought the clinic a malpractice suit. I was also the first woman doctor in the clinic, and one of only a handful of women physicians in semirural Clackamas County. When I finally looked up, Cheryl, our office manager, was standing next to me. She suggested we go into her office. Cheryl was the first one who asked me how I was doing. I told her I wasn't sure, but she seemed reassured that I could answer at all. I didn't know her very well. We were both in our thirties, though she tried to look younger, and I tried to look older. I was a city kid with an *MD* after my name, and she had a diploma from the local high school plus business courses at the community college. I was married without kids and she had kids and an ex. In very different ways, we were both square pegs trying to fit.

Cheryl efficiently made the necessary phone calls. Our malpractice insurance company would have to assign a lawyer to defend me. Our office would have to make copies of the patient's chart for the lawyer. I wanted a copy too. I took it home and read it until late that night, and again and again over the following weeks and months, looking for one thing—what had I done wrong?

The subpoena arrived at my desk on a Tuesday in March. My last note in Helen's chart was from the August before, a visit for chest pain. It was a long note, almost half a page, the longest clinic note in the chart. I reviewed the visits leading up to that last one, reliving each one. I had met her my first year in the practice, in December of the year before she died.

She had gone to the emergency room of our hundred-bed community hospital with chest pain, and one of my senior partners had admitted her for overnight observation. The next day, December 24, was his day off and I was responsible for our patients in the hospital. So I met Helen. Her chest pain had not been a heart attack, according to blood tests overnight. Her pain was gone. But she was, I realized, a time bomb. She had heart disease up and down her family tree, she smoked, and her blood pressure was high. There was probably a heart attack out there with her name on it.

She was friendly with me, smiling and joking in her hospital bed. She was more cheerful than I expected, for someone who had not only gone to an emergency room with chest pain, but had impressed the ER docs enough to admit her. I told her I was glad she hadn't had a heart attack, but that I was worried she was going to, sooner or later. She could save her own life, I said, by quitting smoking and taking care of herself.

She wasn't worried about all that. She wanted to go home and have Christmas with her family.

So I decided to try to get her attention. Her electrocardiogram (EKG) that morning was essentially normal, but not entirely normal. One of the squiggles on the EKG is called a Q wave, a dip down before the up-spike with each heartbeat. Dead sections of heart muscle, permanently damaged by a heart attack, show deep Q waves, as low as the up-spike is high. The normal heart's EKG also has Q waves, but little ones, less than a third the size of the up-spike. And some heart attacks, if they don't damage the full thickness of the heart muscle, don't alter the Q waves at all.

Helen's EKG had normal Q waves, to my relief. But that's not what the computer attached to the EKG machine said. The preliminary interpretation programs that come with EKG machines are hypersensitive, and they read abnormalities where there aren't any. I suppose the reasoning is that oversensitivity is better than undersensitivity. So right up on the top of her EKG, the machine had printed "Probable inferior infarct, old." I had a teaching aid.

I told her she could go home, and that I would prescribe some medicine to block stomach acid because she probably had heartburn. It causes chest pain confusingly similar to the kind of chest pain caused by the heart. Then I showed her the EKG, and told her that, though fortunately her chest pain the night before had not been a heart attack, it looked like she could have had a small heart attack already, some time in the past.

Her eyes got big and quiet. I waited. She said she'd tried to quit smoking before, gotten crabby, and started again. I said it was a hard thing to do, but it paid off. There were medications that prevented heart attacks, which we could talk about in clinic. I seemed to have gotten her attention.

I didn't see her again for a month. She had scheduled her two-week post-hospital visit with my partner who had admitted her to the hospital. She was officially his patient, and he was well known in the community. According to his note in the chart, at that visit she told him that her pain was better, and the way she described it fit the heartburn pattern. My partner scheduled a special X-ray called a barium swallow, which confirmed acid irritation of the stomach. He gave her another acid blocker.

Two weeks later, her time bomb went off. One day in mid-January she came to clinic with bad chest pain. Her acid blocker hadn't helped. She looked terrible. She was frightened and crying. I ran a quick EKG—very abnormal, though still no Q waves—and sent her right up to the hospital. That was her first official heart attack. When I saw her later in the hospital, she was calmer and comfortable, and as friendly as ever, but more serious than I'd ever seen her. She had actually quit smoking a few days before she came to clinic and had started to change her lifestyle. She'd tried to exercise, probably not a good idea for her heart at the time. A few days later, the cardiologists reopened a cholesterol-plugged artery in her heart. After that she could exercise without chest pain and joined a health club. She lost some weight, and stayed off the tobacco. She scheduled most of the rest of her remaining clinic visits with me. I saw her every month or two through the winter, spring, and summer, congratulating her at every visit on her progress, and adjusting her meds for heartburn and high blood pressure. She had another bout of chest pain in the spring, bad enough to stay in the hospital overnight, but that time her morning labs showed no heart attack. She was forty-four years old.

That brought me up to the last visit in the chart, that August. So far I hadn't found what I was looking for—my lethal slip-up must have been in that last visit. The chest pain she had described that day was complicated. But in detail after detail, it fit the pattern of stomach pain rather than heart pain. She had been having it almost around the clock for a couple of weeks. No one could survive a heart in spasm that long—heart pain lasts for a few minutes at a time, off and on. She did not have the nausea, sweats, left arm heaviness, or shortness of breath that she had had with her previous heart attack. Most convincingly, she said she could work out for hours in the gym without pain. She was essentially doing her own treadmill test, and passing. I ran an EKG on her at that last visit, and it was normal—normal for her, that is. Her EKG carried the damage pattern of her first heart attack like a fingerprint, but the EKG that day in August showed nothing new, and even some improvement.

It sure sounded like stomach acid. I gave her samples of a stronger acid blocker, and called her the next day to see if it had worked. When we talked, she said the medication was helping a little. So I switched her to an even stronger acid blocker. And never saw her again.

How else will I someday let a patient down? Most diagnoses are made, not by test results, but by sight, hearing, and touch. (Taste and smell, long used as discriminating diagnostic tools, have fortunately been replaced by chemical analysis.) But every sense I use to search out what's troubling my patient can be mistaken. My eyes, ears, or hands might never have seen a rash like that, heard that kind of cough, or felt a swollen lymph node of that shape before. I might have read something about it, or heard it in a lecture, and forgotten—sometimes it seems that I can't push a new fact into my brain without an old one squirting out. I can also misinterpret what my eyes, ears, or hands are trying to tell me. There are so many ways to hurt people—while trying to help them.

Many of the keys to diagnosis, perhaps most, are embedded in the ways patients tell their stories and describe their symptoms. So many clues, but so many to miss. I might never have heard a patient's voice catch in a certain way before. Or I might suspect but not have the time, or guts, to ask what's going on.

Every way we try to help, if mistaken, can harm instead. The diagnosis can be wrong, or the diagnosis may be too late to do any good. Late diagnosis is often the result of miscommunication, like lost reports or missed phone calls. Overdiagnosis—suspecting or deciding that someone has a disease when they don't—is a mistake too. Overdiagnosis does not seem as irresponsible as missing or delaying a diagnosis, but if someone suffers complications of treatment for a disease they don't have, overdiagnosis can do just as much damage. On the other hand, overdiagnosis is the only way to catch some illnesses that may show only subtle symptoms, like appendicitis: surgeons have a saying that a surgeon who does not take out a few healthy appendixes is missing some sick ones.

I didn't talk to my partners about that final visit with Helen. In medicine we don't talk about our mistakes.

At least, we don't now. Doctors used to—before my time. Way before my time. I didn't know then, as a rookie working out the unspoken rules of the medical fraternity, that doctors had not always kept silent about their own mistakes.

The scientific revolution made the modern medical error possible, beginning about a hundred years ago. Before then, since no one could prove they had the right answers, there were no wrong answers. The life sciences were only born, as real sciences, in the late nineteenth century. Until then every medical sect scrabbling for patients could claim it had the answer: electrical therapy, homegrown herbal therapy, prayer, manipulation, bleeding, purging. None of them could prove the value of its therapy to anyone who didn't already believe in it. Medical mistakes were one practitioner's word against another's.

Before scientific medicine, choosing safe and effective treatment was an iffy business. The standard treatment for dysentery, for example, was purging—inducing vomiting and diarrhea. Anyone who knows even basic first aid must shudder to think of the misery and loss of life induced by this "therapy." But purging remained the authoritative treatment for centuries. Lacking statistical methods—give treatment x to half the patients, y to the other half, and see what happens—therapeutic doctrine rose and fell on the say-so of charismatic professors.

A Kentucky physician, Lunsford Yandell, questioned whether purging was the right way to treat dysentery, in a crisp 1836 case report to his regional medical journal—called the *Transylvania Medical Journal* after that part of Kentucky. He reported on nine patients, their treatment, and his results. He administered purging to most of them, and several died, one of them a six-year-old boy. One woman refused his treatment, took broth instead, and lived. The doctor described each case, one by one, in the cold language of scholars. He ended with the unusual conclusion that purging, the established professional treatment for dysentery, had been "utterly futile" for these patients.

Hidden in family letters was the reason these cases led him to openly challenge tradition: the woman who refused his treatment and lived was his wife. The six-year-old boy who died was their son.

Much later, the laboratory would prove some answers right and others wrong. Breakthroughs in microbiology, infectious disease, biochemistry, and laboratory technology changed diagnosis and treatment from matters of opinion to matters of cold, hard fact. The scientific revolution of the nineteenth century created medical error in the modern sense: mistakes became deviations from known facts or proven standards of care.

And physicians openly discussed their failings in meetings and in new medical journals, to ask for critique, so that colleagues could learn from each other's mistakes. It is hard to imagine now, but in the first years of the twentieth century Harvey Cushing, the founder of neurosurgery, frankly discussed his own surgical mistakes in print. He published critical descriptions of his own cases, both successes and failures, in medical journals, writing, for example, in 1903 about a patient who improved after brain surgery to remove a blood clot. On the first day after surgery: "At an ill-advised moment . . . the dressing was removed, . . . and the scalp sutured in place . . . This misjudged procedure evidently turned the balance . . . At midnight, three and a half days after the operation, death occurred." Despite the passive verbs, this surgeon is describing his own actions. He does not describe his feelings, which we can only imagine. Cushing published one more self-critical series of cases in 1905, but medical publication was becoming more circumspect. Mistakes were going underground.

Professional silence hardened in the United States with the burgeoning of malpractice cases in the 1900s. Malpractice lawsuits were rare in the 1800s. In the first decades of the twentieth century, however, the legal profession invented the contingency fee—the client paid the attorney only if he won—which meant that patients could sue without financial risk. Malpractice numbers exploded. In 1935 the *New England Journal of Medicine* reported 20,000 lawsuits in the previous five years. The medical profession closed ranks. Journal articles advised a new professional etiquette: never criticize another physician in front of a patient and, if sued, don't talk about it, especially not to the patient.

I wouldn't be writing about medical errors, and you wouldn't be reading about them, if not for David Hilfiker. Through most of the twentieth century, medical tradition and custom hushed up our mistakes. Hilfiker made a terrible mistake. But instead of crawling under the carpet, he lifted it up in the very public pages of the *New England Journal of Medicine.* In 1984, when I was a second-year medical student, he wrote a searching, taboo-smashing personal essay about how it felt to make a mistake.

Hilfiker, a family doctor in rural Minnesota, told a story about a family he knew as friends, neighbors, and patients. He had delivered their first baby, and they came to him when the mom felt pregnant again. But her pregnancy test was negative, several times, over several weeks. She still felt pregnant, and on exam her uterus was slightly enlarged as if in early pregnancy. But those negative tests said something was wrong. It seemed that the fetus had died, but not yet been miscarried. Hilfiker shared his friends' sadness, and he recommended waiting a few weeks for the miscarriage to take its course.

Weeks later, she had still not miscarried, her uterus was still slightly enlarged, and she still felt pregnant—but yet another pregnancy test was negative. Hilfiker recommended the standard treatment, a D and C, dilation and curettage, to clean out the dead tissue before it became infected.

During the procedure he realized something was terribly wrong. He wrote: "This morning there is considerably more blood than usual . . . The body parts I remove are much larger than I had expected, considering when the fetus died."

Harvey Cushing's self-critical publication about his error left his own feelings out of it, to spotlight the details of surgical technique for generations of students. Hilfiker gives his readers just enough surgical detail to orient them in the story, so that he can illuminate and dissect his feelings, the true pathology of the story, so familiar and yet so unexamined for his readers: "I suppress the rising panic . . .

In a daze I . . . try to tell Russ and Barb as much as I know, without telling them all that I suspect."

The facts of modern medicine are now determined objectively. But the spiritual and ethical content of the medical life is passed down from professor to student in much the same way that the rules for treating dysentery were passed down to Lunsford Yandell in the 1830s. Like Yandell, Hilfiker reports on the tradition he accepted from his teachers and now finds utterly futile.

In the large centers where doctors are trained, . . . a mistake is first whispered about in the halls, as if it were a sin. The medical profession simply seems to have no place for its mistakes.

The only real answer for guilt is spiritual confession, restitution, and absolution. Yet within the structure of modern medicine there is simply no place for this spiritual healing.

The letters in response broke all records at the *New England Journal of Medicine*. The vehemence of the letters was also unprecedented, ranging from sneering denunciations of Hilfiker's incompetence to effusive praise of his personal courage.

After Hilfiker broke the silence in 1984, research on medical error began to trickle into medical journals. The researchers had to begin with the basic questions: How many? What types? How much damage is done? It's difficult to analyze medical mistakes, however, because the typical reaction to making a mistake—withdrawal into self-flagellating shame—confounds data-gathering.

Researchers looking at how doctors deal with mistakes find that many don't talk to anyone at all. In a 1992 study, a psychologist interviewed physicians about their experience of medical error. Some physicians in the study said they feared being "found out" as incompetent after making a mistake. I can still remember that feeling in my stomach, looking down at my subpoena. Many of the interviewees feared ostracism if their mistake were known: "I hear doctors talk about other doctors. I figure that behind my back they'll probably say the same kinds of things about me."

In med school in the 1980s, my classmates and I obsessed about the infinite number of mistakes we might someday make. But if we really did make a mistake, or observed someone else's mistake, we would not have known what to do. The curriculum faced other uncomfortable subjects—like how to talk to patients about death or sex—but it didn't go near that one.

It can be hard to go on after making a mistake that harms someone. A few years after his essay appeared, Hilfiker, still a wounded healer, left his small town practice to serve in an AIDS hospice in a large city.

I didn't talk to my partners, but I started sending a lot more people to the hospital for chest pain. I no longer trusted my teachers or mentors or textbooks to tell me the difference between heartburn and a bad heart. Real human bodies weren't obliged to follow rules in books.

I knew Helen had died sometime after seeing me that August, but the subpoena didn't say when, or how. I didn't learn what had killed her until I attended the pretrial deposition of Helen's adult daughter, three months after my subpoena arrived.

Helen's daughter lived with her, and found her in bed one morning, ten days after that last appointment with me. Helen had died in her sleep.

Oh.

That meant that what had probably killed Helen was her heart suddenly jumping into a bad rhythm, a rhythm that didn't pump blood forward. Heart muscle damaged by a previous heart attack is "irritable" and can fall into a strange rhythm at any time. We didn't then, and still don't, have any good way of predicting whose damaged hearts are more likely to do that, or when.

What killed Helen is called sudden cardiac death. There's one good drug that keeps an irritable heart in its proper rhythm, lidocaine, but it can only be given intravenously, with careful monitoring. The story of heart-rhythm drug development is a search for a safe oral equivalent of lidocaine that patients can take at home. So far, pills to prevent sudden cardiac death are mostly not very effective, pleasant, or safe.

Oh.

Helen had apparently died of a form of heart disease that I couldn't have diagnosed, predicted, or prevented. Maybe I hadn't screwed up after all.

Maybe I was, after all, good enough to do this. Not perfect, not by a long shot. But good enough. Good enough to be a doctor.

I wasn't prepared for that.

Learning from my subpoena that I wasn't good enough to be a doctor hurt. But it was no surprise. It was like the other shoe dropping, a constant theme of medical training. Learning that I hadn't done anything wrong, at least not this time—I didn't know what to make of that.

I finally talked to my partners. One of them told me about a patient of his who regularly experienced four different kinds of chest pain: angina from her heart, pleurisy from her lungs, arthritis from her ribs, and heartburn from her stomach. I learned that mine was not, after all, the first malpractice suit in the clinic, and that the senior partners I looked up to had been equally devastated by their experiences.

I knew Helen's family and her lawyer couldn't possibly know what medicine could, and couldn't, do for her. No one reviews malpractice lawsuits for scientific validity before they're filed. If I were Helen's family, I might have sued, too. They had never met me—unlike the majority of our patients, Helen never brought anyone with her to clinic. I felt sorry for her daughter. Her mom was dead, and I hadn't stopped what killed her—of course it was my fault. I also knew that, whatever the facts, and whatever the legal process decided, I would always be responsible for Helen's death in their eyes. And if the legal process went against me, if the jury decided I was guilty of medical negligence in her death, others would consider me responsible for her death too. My name would go on state and national lists of doctors who had been sued for malpractice and lost. I would be named a bad doctor.

The trial approached, and it mattered to me as a matter of honor. I prepared for it as a performance. My character would be the conscientious, boringly consistent, and compulsively thorough but compassionate young physician. Actually, that is me. But in clinic, with patients, I had always tried to seem more relaxed and casual, because all that compulsiveness made people nervous. For the trial I bought a brown leather purse. The purple fanny pack I had carried since residency didn't give quite the right image. I bought a gray wool blazer, and chose similar band-collared, light-colored blouses and conservative skirts to wear with it every day. I wore my long wavy hair back in a barrette every day. I didn't know how many days of trial I would have to plan costumes for.

My lawyer said I was lucky to have the case come to trial in less than a year; the average wait used to be three years. The trial took ten days, at the redbrick county courthouse a few blocks from the clinic.

There were some surprises.

Helen had quit smoking. But I learned that her family and friends hadn't— why should they? I knew that research showed cigarette smoke increased the risk of abnormal heart rhythms. After the trial I started asking my patients, not just whether they smoked and if they were ready to think about quitting, but whether anyone else was exposing them to secondhand smoke.

I also heard another side of Helen's story from that last visit—the part about working out in that gym for hours without chest pain. Her daughter and a friend who went to the gym with them testified on the stand that Helen could only stay on those exercise machines a few minutes before she had to stop and rest until the chest pain went away.

She lied to me. Perhaps that was fair. I had lied to her only a few months before, trying to save her life. Patients and their doctors lie to each other for all sorts of reasons.

The reason Helen lied, I think, is that she was playing a role, the role of the good patient. She was telling me what she thought I wanted to hear. Maybe she wanted to hear me congratulate her again on how well she was doing.

It's not just her: all my patients are acting. By the time I walk into that exam room, they have written a whole script, with heroes, villains, and lines for me. Every clinic visit is a scene. I have to figure out on the fly what my cues are, and whether my playwright on the exam table is an honest one. The power of the patient-physician relationship, which is gradually going extinct in the era of managed care, is that when patient and physician know each other, they can stop acting.

But I didn't see through Helen's performance. That was the mistake I made. That was my negligence. It has taken me a lot of miles since medical school, walking in suffering people's moccasins, to hear the ways patients bend the truth, and to see the truths they can't face. I believed her. I don't know if I could have done anything about it if I had seen through her, but that will always be with me. How many other cheerful lies and half-truths have I missed?

I "won" the case and went back to work. I hadn't seen my patients for a week and a half, and there was a lot of catching up to do.

I say it was my first malpractice suit. There hasn't been a second—yet—but I don't want to get overconfident.

"Missing" is the winner of
The Creative Nonfiction *Silence Kills* Best Essay Award.

Merilee D. Karr is a health and science journalist, family physician, playwright, and dramaturge. She has published in the *Journal of Irreproducible Results*, *JAMA*, *Metroscape*, and *Seattle Weekly* and pitched story ideas to the *Star Trek* TV series. Her response to managed care is leaving medicine to write about it. She is an adjunct assistant professor in family medicine at Oregon Health and Sciences University and a student in the Nonfiction Writing program at Portland State University. She is working on a book about cultural obstacles to patient safety.

REFERENCES

Christiansen, John F., Wendy Levinson, and Patrick M. Dunn. "The heart of darkness: The impact of perceived mistakes on physicians." *Journal of General Internal Medicine* 7 (1992): 424–31. Interviews of physicians on attitudes toward mistakes.

Hilfiker, David. "Facing our mistakes." *New England Journal of Medicine* 310 (1984): 118–22.

Pinkus, Rosa Lynn. "Mistakes as a social construct: An historical approach." *Kennedy Institute of Ethics Journal* 11, no. 2 (2001): 117–33. On early twentieth-century discussion of medical errors by Cushing, and their subsequent suppression.

Stowe, Steven M. "Seeing themselves at work: Physicians and the case narrative in the mid-19th-century American South." In *Sickness and health in America*, ed. Judith Walzer Leavitt and Ron Numbers. On Lunsford Yandell.

Mrs. Kelly

Paul Austin

"It's not that bad." Mr. Kelly smiled. "I'm not even hurting now." He was a forty-two-year-old house painter who'd been having intermittent chest pain for two days. Three wires ran from under his patient gown to the monitor in the corner, where a fine green line bounced with every beat of his heart.

His wife shifted in her chair. A disposal box for contaminated needles jutted from the wall, next to her head. She leaned away from it, as if she wanted to scoot her chair over. A stainless steel supply rack hemmed her in on the other side.

"It was just a nagging little pain." He gestured toward his chest. His finger-nails were square and stubby, trimmed close. His nails glowed pink against the white paint stuck to his cuticles.

"How long did the pain last?" I asked.

"I don't know, Doc." He looked at his wife, then back to me. "About ten, fifteen minutes."

"Did you tell him about your arm hurting?" Mrs. Kelly was a thin woman. She sat with her feet tucked beneath the chair and her hands held tightly together in her lap.

"It didn't hurt that bad." He rolled his left shoulder. "I mighta pulled it at work. You know, moving ladders and all."

Mrs. Kelly shook her head.

I asked him about the cardiac risk factors: he didn't know his cholesterol, he smoked about a pack a day, and his father had had a heart attack when he was in his late fifties. I wrote orders for the standard workup: EKG, cardiac enzymes, chest X-ray, and routine labs. "When the results come back, we'll talk." I went to see my next patient.

The EKG was done promptly. Normal. The blood work and chest X-rays were normal too. But I had been practicing for ten years, and knew that in the evaluation of chest pain the symptoms and risk factors are more important than the tests.

During a myocardial infarction—a heart attack—heart cells die, releasing enzymes into the blood. Early on, the level might not reach the threshold of "positive." We check subsequent levels to catch any rise that may occur over time. The safest thing to do would be to admit Mr. Kelly overnight.

Mr. Kelly didn't have a physician, so I called the on-call doctor to arrange for an overnight admission and serial enzymes.

In training, interns and residents work incessantly. I remembered being on call, and to a bleary-eyed intern who was hoping to sneak off and take a nap at 3:00 in the morning, no page from the ER was good news. It didn't mean that I was getting the opportunity to help someone, or that I was getting a case I could learn from. It just meant that I was getting screwed out of the few hours of sleep I'd been hoping to steal.

When a patient needed to be admitted to the hospital where I trained, the senior resident went to the ER and checked on the patient. If an admission was unavoidable, the senior called the intern, who came down to do the history and physical and write the admission orders. If there was some doubt as to the necessity of an admission, the senior resident might put up a fight with the ER attending physician, and try to talk him into sending the patient home. Some of the senior residents never questioned the ER attending. We called them "sieves," because they let everyone in. Those who consistently argued against admissions were called "walls." "Sieves" were despised by interns. "Walls" were worshipped; they shielded their interns by thinking of fifty different reasons every patient could be discharged. And they just seemed smarter than the "sieves."

This attitude is understandable when you consider the hallucinatory, sleepless fog of residency and the fact that residents are young, still in training. Most physicians gradually outgrow this attitude as they work easier hours and take on more responsibility for patient care. Some, though, even years out of training, seem to take pride in being a "wall," sending people home from the ER. George Packard was one of those guys.

He was the doctor on call for patients without a primary care physician, so I called him. He'd been in practice for years, and he was a "wall." Proud of it. Had a cocky little walk he did when he discharged a patient from the ER. When we called him about one of his own patients, he'd try to talk us into sending him or her home. When he was on call for unassigned patients, he argued even more stubbornly. I wasn't looking forward to the call.

George returned the page, and we talked.

"Sounds like he could go home."

"I don't know, George." I stared across the ER at a drunk who was leaning farther and farther across the side rail of his stretcher. Blood dripped slowly from a laceration on his forehead. I covered the phone's mouthpiece. "Someone help that guy in Room 8," I yelled. "He's about to fall." One of the health care techs strolled into the room and pushed the drunk back on the stretcher.

"The guy has a strong family history and he's a smoker," I said into the phone. "Stoic guy, may be in denial. I think he's real, and he needs to come in."

"You think everyone needs to come in."

"This guy has a good story." The drunk had his head over the side rail and was looking at something on the floor.

"You're saying you think he's having a heart attack?"

"I'm saying he could have a plaque that hasn't ruptured yet."

"Didn't you just tell me he had a normal EKG and negative enzymes?"

We both knew Mr. Kelly could be having a heart attack and initially have normal studies. That's why we admit patients for serial tests. "I don't know what to tell you, George." I shook my head. "Guy's dad had an MI in his fifties, he smokes a pack a day, and his pain is typical of ischemia."

"With a normal EKG, and negative enzymes after two days of intermittent pain. If anything was going to be positive, it already would've been. You know that."

"I think he needs to be admitted." I wished we had an equation we could apply to the problem. So many points for this risk factor, so many points for the other. But there isn't one. It all comes down to a judgment call, based on a few risk factors and very subjective symptoms. Pain versus pressure, discomfort versus pain. Is the patient exaggerating or minimizing his symptoms?

"I'd be glad to squeeze him in at the office, first thing in the morning. Do an accelerated outpatient workup."

"I don't think he should go home tonight."

"Do you know how many hundreds of patients with bullshit chest pain we admit for every patient who has real disease? Or have any idea how many billions we spend every year on these worthless admissions? How much 'covering your ass' costs?"

"I'd love to talk about that sometime, but not right now." The drunk had given up whatever he'd been trying to do, and lay with his head half off the stretcher, passed out. "And we're not talking about 'covering my ass.' We're talking about a guy who needs to be admitted to rule out MI."

"If I come in, I'm just going to send him home."

"That'll be your decision."

"You're going to make the patient wait another two hours?" George's voice scaled upward with incredulity. "Just for me to come in and send him home? I'm offering to see him first thing in the morning. That's only fourteen hours from now."

Two paramedics stood in the hallway with an asthmatic patient on a stretcher, waiting for the charge nurse to tell them where to put him. He opened his mouth like a fish with each inspiration, the muscles in his neck tightening into cords with the effort. His skin was gray, and shiny with sweat.

"George, the guy needs to come in."

"It's up to you." George was probably shrugging on the other end. "I'll come in, but it sounds like he can go home."

We didn't have a bed for the asthmatic, and he was too sick to stay in the hall. No point in tying up a bed with Mr. Kelly if George was going to send him home. "You'll see my guy first thing in the morning?"

"Glad to." George's voice warmed up.

Mr. Kelly and his wife looked at me when I walked into the cubicle. "Your EKG and labs are normal."

Mr. Kelly smiled, looked at his wife, then back to me. He waited.

"I think we can let you go home."

"Great." Mr. Kelly grinned and gave me a thumbs-up. His wife looked down at her hands.

"I've spoken with Dr. Packard, the doctor on call. He'll see you in the morning, in his office."

His wife didn't look up. I got the feeling she wanted her husband to stay, but she didn't say anything.

"I think you'll be fine, but if you have any chest pain, come back immediately." I waited for them to respond. If either of them objected, I could call Packard back and tell him they were balking at going home. Mrs. Kelly didn't look up. Of course, I could call Packard back anyway, and tell him to get himself to the ER and see the patient. Let *him* send the guy home.

I didn't.

Joanne, the charge nurse, had pulled a different patient into the hall to make room for the asthmatic.

Lisa, one of the nurses, was slapping the back of the asthmatic's hand to find a vein in which to start an IV. "The line EMS put in blew." She didn't look up from her task. "I went ahead and started another breathing treatment."

"Good." I nodded to the patient, then, with my stethoscope, listened to the tight, high-pitched wheezing sounds of air barely moving in and out of his lungs. "You sound tight," I said to the man.

He nodded.

"Let's give him Solumedrol," I said to Lisa.

"Got it in my pocket." She looked up. "Can you hand me some tape?"

I tore two thin strips of tape and handed them to her.

"Thanks." She taped the IV in place. "There." She looked to me. "Portable X-ray?"

"Yup." With good nurses, an ER doc can get a lot done, just by saying "yup." I saw Mr. Kelly and his wife walking toward the exit. I wanted to call out, "Wait, let's check another EKG." But a repeat EKG would probably be normal too, and I would've felt foolish asking him to stay after I'd discharged him. And I'd arranged follow-up for the next morning. He'd be OK for fourteen hours.

"Paul," Lisa called, "this guy's looking sick."

I turned to the asthmatic, and forgot Mr. Kelly.

The next day when I started my shift, Joe, one of the other ER doctors, was sitting in the dictation room. He was a runner, and looked like it. Tall, bony guy with broad shoulders and a skinny butt. He looked up from the chart he was working on. "Paul, you remember a guy named Kelly?"

My stomach felt queasy. "Guy with chest pain?"

"Yeah." Joe looked up from the chart he was holding. "He came back, about 4:30 in the morning. Cardiac arrest."

I sat.

"You OK?"

"Yeah." I felt prickles in my scalp and down the back of my neck. I glanced at the trash can, afraid I might vomit. "He'd been having chest pain off and on. Didn't have any while he was here."

"I worked the code for at least thirty minutes before I called it."

Mr. Kelly was dead.

Joe adjusted the stethoscope draped around his neck. "I looked over his EKG and labs from when you'd seen him. They were normal."

"I know." I'd sent Mr. Kelly home, and now he was dead.

"It's gonna happen." Joe shook his head. "We can't admit every single chest pain that comes in. I would've done the same thing."

I still wanted to puke. "I had a bad feeling about him when I let him go."

Joe shrugged. "I sent home a guy last year. Came back a couple of hours later with ST segments like Mount Everest." He was describing a classic EKG pattern of a heart attack.

"Did your guy make it?"

"Yeah," Joe said, "but that's not the point. I'd sent him home. I was just lucky."

He was trying to help me feel better. Every doctor has had a patient die as the result of a wrong judgment call, or a brief lapse of attention. It's inevitable when fallible people make mortal decisions. There are people who'll say, "This should never happen." And they're absolutely right. It shouldn't.

• • •

I struggled through the shift, oppressed by the knowledge that I'd sent Mr. Kelly home, and that he'd died. Maybe if I'd paid attention to his wife, her unease would've prompted me to ask more questions. Maybe I would have learned something to make me insist on his admission. But I'd looked Mr. Kelly in the eye and told him I thought he'd be OK, even though I had misgivings. I'd not paid enough attention to an intuition, an uneasy feeling, and there hadn't been enough hard data to convince George Packard to come in. I'd trusted his judgment over mine.

In lectures, seminars, and magazine articles, malpractice lawyers tell you never, never, never to discuss a potential malpractice case. With anyone. The other side will ask if you discussed it, and ask for a list of names. Then they'll interview people until they find one who remembers your admitting a mistake. In one class I listened to on cassette tape, the speaker told about a doctor who'd confided in his wife about a mistake he'd made. Before the case went to court, the doctor and his wife went through an acrimonious divorce. In the malpractice trial, the ex-wife took the stand against him with a vengeance. The class had roared with laughter at the poor schmuck's bad luck. You don't discuss the case, and you never, ever, apologize. To the malpractice lawyers, "I'm sorry" is just another way to say "I'm guilty."

The shift moved slowly, like a bad dream. Finally, it was over. Before I left, I copied Mr. Kelly's phone number down on a scrap of paper.

When I got home, everyone was asleep. I wanted to talk with my wife, Sally. But she was sleeping soundly, so I went downstairs and turned on the TV. A tall, handsome attorney with a very good toupee was on the screen. His voice was deep, and caring: "If you, or anyone in your family, has been injured by a doctor or a hospital, call me." A 1–800 number flashed on the screen. "We'll get the money you deserve." He somehow managed to mix enthusiasm with sadness in his voice. I vaguely wondered if Mrs. Kelly was at home alone, watching the same ad.

"What if she is?" I asked out loud. I clicked off the TV. "She may want to give dip-shit a call." I went to the kitchen, got a beer, and went out on the front porch and sat on the steps. Two large magnolia trees shaded me from the streetlight. Mrs. Kelly was probably awake, too. Maybe sitting on her front porch looking out into the night, stunned by the emptiness she faced.

The next morning I was off duty. After the kids were in school, I told Sally. She listened to the whole story.

"Paul, there's no way you could've known he was going to die."

"His story was good enough to buy an admission."

"No one's perfect." She shook her head. "I know it makes your job scary, but everyone is going to make mistakes."

"Yeah, but not like this." I rinsed my coffee cup. "Missing a fracture, or a UTI, stuff like that, sure, you're going to miss a few of them. But sending a guy home to die?" I felt the pain continue to build, of all places, in my chest. Maybe if I cried, I'd feel better.

"You didn't send anyone home to die." Sally sounded a little irritated. "You evaluated him, and made a decision." Simple as that. "No one expects you to be perfect." She hadn't seen the ad last night on TV.

"Even if I'd admitted him, he probably would have died."

"That's true." Sally nodded.

I leaned against the kitchen counter, my back to the sun coming through the kitchen window. "Must've been a huge MI, to have killed him so quickly." I needed to believe Mr. Kelly would've died even if I'd admitted him, because nothing in my experience had prepared me for feeling so guilty. Up to the moment I'd heard about Mr. Kelly, the possibility I could make an error of that magnitude had remained an abstraction, a theoretical possibility with no grounding in personal experience. I'd been trained well and I was careful. I thought that if I was vigilant enough, I could practice indefinitely without seriously hurting anyone.

I sat at the kitchen table, replaying the scene of Mr. Kelly and his wife shuffling down the hall in the ER, wishing I could rewind it all and call out to tell them that I'd changed my mind, that I'd admit him to the hospital.

The phone rang. It was Ken, one of the guys in our group. He's been an ER doc for twenty years. He has graying hair, a calm voice, and never seems to hurry. Even when the ER is rocking, Ken looks like he just strolled off the golf course. I don't know how he does it: each month we get a report on how many patients we see each hour, and Ken's numbers are consistently good, but he rarely seems perturbed, and I've never seen him look rushed.

"Paul," he said, "I was going to drop by if you're around."

"Sure," I said. "You know our address?"

"Yeah," he said, "I'm about a block away." Car phone.

"OK." I hung up. "That was Ken," I said to Sally. "He's coming over."

"It'll be good to talk with him," she said. "Why don't I go work in the yard some, give you guys some space." She stepped forward for a quick hug, then walked out the back door.

I went to the bathroom, then looked at my face in the mirror, hoping I didn't look as vulnerable as I felt. I also hoped I wasn't in trouble with the hospital, or the group of ER docs I worked with. I felt vaguely nauseated again.

Ken knocked on the door, and I let him in. He followed me back to the kitchen.

"I was just about to make a pot of coffee," I said.

"Sounds good." He sat in the chair at the end of the kitchen table.

"Are you here about Mr. Kelly?" I rinsed the basket of the coffee maker and put in a clean filter.

"Yeah."

I turned to look at Ken. "I feel terrible."

"You should," he said. "The man died."

I turned back around, hoping I hadn't outwardly flinched. Neither of us spoke as I silently counted the scoops of coffee. I dropped the scoop back into the coffee jar, and closed it.

"And good doctors," Ken continued, "are bothered when one of their patients dies."

Ken still thought I was a good doctor? I felt a wave of gratitude and relief. I put the coffee pot under the basket and punched the button to start the brewing. "I feel like I killed the guy."

"Whoa," Ken said. "Back up a minute. You didn't kill anybody. You're not even sure of the cause of death."

"Guy comes in with chest pain, comes back dead?" I turned to face Ken. "Not exactly rocket science."

"OK, say the man died of a heart attack. No matter how careful, how smart, or how compulsive you are, eventually you're going to make a mistake."

"Yeah, I know." I sat in the chair at the other end of the table. "Missing something really obscure, or something so rare no one else would've picked it up either." I shrugged. "To me, that wouldn't be so hard to live with. But sending home a patient who is having a heart attack?"

"Paul, we can't admit every single patient who comes in with chest pain." Ken shook his head. "It's impossible. The hospital wouldn't hold them all." Ken looked over his shoulder at the coffee pot. "I think it's ready."

I got up and poured us each a cup.

"I'm just glad it was you, and not me."

"Thanks, pal." I tried to chuckle.

"What can I say?" He sipped his coffee. "Luck of the draw who picks up what chart."

"Ken, have you ever sent someone home and they came back dead?"

He carefully set his cup down, and gently rapped the table with his knuckles. "Knock on wood."

I wrapped my hands around the mug of coffee to feel the warmth.

"But Paul," he said, "It's going to happen. It's like driving a car. No matter how careful you are, someday you're going to glance down at the radio to change stations, look up, and there's a car right in front of you. You've had a clean driving record for thirty years, you're a model citizen, and boom. You've plowed into some little old lady's Cadillac." He shook his head. "I'm not saying you made a mistake with this guy, but even good drivers have accidents."

"How do you do it?"

"Do what?"

"Keep on making life-and-death decisions, knowing that you're fallible."

"Paul, I don't make life-and-death decisions." He carefully put his coffee cup on the table. "I make medical decisions." He gave a slight shrug. "I work as carefully as I can, but it's not up to me, who lives and who dies."

I stared at Ken's face.

"That's God's department."

OK.

"Do you know what happens when a patient dies?"

"Yeah," I said. "The doc feels like shit."

"That's not what I mean." Ken looked away, then looked back. "We can describe, down at the molecular level, what happens when a cell dies: membranes break down, oxidative phosphorylation fails, hydrogen ions accumulate in the cytoplasm, all that stuff. But do we really know why people die?"

I couldn't see what he was getting at.

"Say someone comes in with a pulmonary embolism. We understand the pathophysiology: hypoxia, hypotension, acidosis, etcetera." He paused. "And we know how to intervene."

I nodded.

"But when a patient dies, what happens?" He raised his eyebrows. "I mean, one moment they're alive, and the next, they're not. You've felt it. We all have. Something's happened, and we don't know what it is. Sure, we can trace out the failures of the circulatory system, and we can get EEGs for brain activity." Ken shook his head. "But the fundamental thing of death itself is something we still don't understand."

"So?" I said.

"So, I look at each EKG as carefully as I can, and interview each patient as carefully as I can, and I make decisions as carefully as I can. Then I do my job and I let God do his." Ken held his hands out, palms up. "How can we possibly claim the credit for success, or take the blame for failure, in a process we don't really understand?"

I shrugged.

"Paul, you and I both know you did your best for that man." Ken shook his head. "That's all any of us can do."

When I'd first started working in Durham, I'd been surprised by how much I liked talking with Ken. In so many ways, we're polar opposites: He's a conservative Republican. He wears knit shirts and khaki pants on his days off. He belongs to two country clubs: one here in Durham, one at his beach house. He thinks Rush Limbaugh is smart. I'd always thought of Ken as someone with useful answers to questions about buying stocks or avoiding taxes, but I hadn't thought he'd be the one to say something that would help me deal with the unexpected death of a patient.

Ken stood, and took his coffee mug to the kitchen counter. "Give my love to Sally."

"I will. Tell Barbara I said hey."

Ken rinsed his cup, and left it in the sink. "You're going to feel bad for a while," Ken said. "That's OK. Just keep feeling bad. You'll eventually feel better."

We walked to the front door.

"When do you work again?"

"Day after tomorrow."

"See you then." He stuck out his hand. "Paul, you're a good doctor."

"Thanks." We shook hands and he left. I felt my eyes fill, and hoped Ken hadn't noticed. It must've been awkward for him to come by and talk with me, and I didn't want to go all gushy on him. I felt as though being a good father, or a good husband, or a good man was a hollow success if I wasn't a good doctor as well. Sure, he's a great guy, just don't go to him if you have an emergency. I was relieved that Ken thought I was a good doctor. I just wished I could agree with him.

After Ken drove away, I walked outside. It was a bright, sunny day, but Mr. Kelly was still dead. I sat in a wicker chair and wondered if I could get some relief by praying. A Quaker upbringing had taught me to pray silently. I started that way, but felt a need for something more physical and real than closing my eyes and thinking about God. "Lord, you know I'm not much of a Christian. I doubt. I curse. And I think about sex all the time. You know that. And you know I'm too quick to laugh at tragic stuff if it's funny." I took a deep breath. "You know all that. And you know I sent Mr. Kelly home. And he died." I blew my nose into my fingers. "I don't know if it counts as an honest mistake or a sin." I wiped my hand on my jeans, and looked out at the street. The sun was still bright, the porch was still in the shade. A woman walked past, a dog tugging on a leash. I closed my eyes. "God, forgive me. And be with Mrs. Kelly, and their kids, if they have any." I took a deep breath. "Comfort them. And let them know I did the best I could, and I'm sorry." I opened my eyes. No change.

Maybe I should talk with Karen, or James, I thought. They're our pastors, at the Pilgrim United Church of Christ. When Sally and I had kids, we started going to the Pilgrim UCC in Durham. The folks there seem like Unitarians, only less embarrassed to be called Christians. We went to Sunday school and church almost every Sunday I was off duty. Matthew, my Sunday school teacher, was a constitutional law professor at Duke. Worked with Janet Reno and Al Gore on some legal issues. I felt lucky to discuss Christianity with such smart people, because so much of Christianity in the South seems anti-intellectual—TV preachers sputtering about sin and pleading for money, telephone numbers flashing on the screen. I've always felt like a second-rate Christian, insufficiently saved, with inadequate fervor. At the same time, I feel the Bible drawing me back, particularly the four Gospels. I believe there are answers there. And a model of grace. A model of how I can live.

I wiped my hand on my pants again, then went inside and called Karen. She said I could come over right then. I changed jeans, splashed my face, and drove to our church, a brick building that's mostly roofline, tucked in among a thick stand of trees that shields it from the traffic on the street.

When I knocked on her office door, Karen said, "Come in." She walked from behind her desk, and gestured to an upholstered chair. Another chair faced mine. She pulled it toward mine a little, and sat. "Are you OK?"

"Yeah, basically." I told her the story. "I feel so bad. So guilty." I looked at the floor, then back to Karen. "You know, in the Bible, it says if we want God to forgive us for something we did to someone else, we should first ask that person's forgiveness? Something about leaving the gift on the altar, straightening out the problem, then coming back."

Karen nodded.

"I want to call Mrs. Kelly and tell her I'm sorry."

"It'll be a tough call to make," Karen was looking me in the eyes.

"Not as hard as walking around feeling as bad as I do now."

"Maybe."

"I don't know if I'm wanting to call Mrs. Kelly to make her feel better, or to make myself feel better."

"And?" Karen's face seemed to say that either reason would be OK.

"It's probably a little of both."

Karen waited.

"Do I have the right to call Mrs. Kelly, just to make myself feel better?"

"Paul," Karen's voice scaled down several tones. "It's all right for you to want forgiveness." She shook her head. "God doesn't want you to carry guilt and pain every step of your life."

I didn't feel anything in my chest loosen up, or feel any burden lighten. But I caught a glimmer of the possibility. I thanked her.

When I got home, I looked at the phone number on the scrap of paper.

Sally walked into the kitchen. She was sweaty from mowing the yard. "How did it go with Karen?"

"I'd hoped I would feel better."

Sally smiled. "You look a little better."

"I think I'll call Mrs. Kelly." I walked to the sink and got a glass of water. "Tell her I'm sorry."

Sally hugged me from behind. I could feel the damp of her shirt.

I sat the water on the counter, and turned to return the hug. Mrs. Kelly didn't have a husband to hug any more. Damn.

"If I call her, and it goes to court, they'll make a big deal about me calling her to apologize."

Sally shrugged.

"If the award goes past my malpractice coverage, it could come out of our pockets."

"So what. It'll probably never happen." She shrugged again. "And if it does: Fuck 'em."

If nothing else, I'd married well.

Sally pulled back to look at me. "Call her. You may feel better." She hugged me again. "I'll be on the front porch."

• • •

Mrs. Kelly picked up the phone on the third ring.

"This is Paul Austin. I'm the doctor who took care of your husband the first time he came to the emergency room."

"Oh."

"I'm calling to say I'm sorry." I paused. "I'm sorry your husband died."

She didn't answer.

"Mrs. Kelly?"

"I'm here."

I waited. "If you have any questions, or concerns . . ."

There was another pause. "Why did you send my husband home?"

The question thumbed me in the chest. "I thought he would be OK." I took a breath. "I was wrong. And I'm sorry."

She didn't answer.

I waited.

She didn't say anything.

I looked down at the crumbs on the floor. "If there's anything you want to say to me . . ." I winced at the accusations she might unleash, but held a glimmer of hope she'd say she forgave me.

"I've got nothing to say to you right now."

I gave her my home phone number, and told her if she ever had anything to say, or any other questions, I'd be glad to talk with her.

We hung up.

I didn't feel any better. And it seemed Mrs. Kelly didn't feel any better either.

I walked out to the front porch.

Sally looked up from her novel. "How did it go?"

I sat in the chair next to her. "She didn't have anything to say to me."

Sally closed her novel, keeping her place with her finger.

"I didn't really expect her to flat-out forgive me, but I'd hoped for something." Glints of sunlight reflected off the hard, waxy leaves of the magnolia tree in front of the porch. I could barely make out the pitted gray bark of the trunk through the dark openings between the leaves. "Some human contact."

"It's early." Sally patted my knee.

"Did I call too soon?" I felt my dismay grow heavier, like a rain-soaked coat. Had I added to Mrs. Kelly's pain, just to ease my own? Every place I turned, I was screwing up.

"Probably not." Sally shook her head. "But who knows when you should've called? She might've been sitting at her kitchen table just now, wondering why the ER doctor hadn't even bothered to call." Sally turned in her chair to face me. "At least now she knows her husband was important to the doctor."

"Yeah, I guess."

"You guess? Paul, you've done everything you could—you saw the guy, did all the tests, thought about it, and told him to come back if he had more pain." She held up a finger with each point. "Nobody's perfect."

"I know." Every single thing she'd said was true.

But Mr. Kelly was still dead.

Paul Austin has worked in emergency care for thirty years, first as a firefighter and now as a physician. His book about the way his job almost destroyed his family will be published by W. W. Norton in the spring of 2008. His essays have been published or are forthcoming in *Gettysburg Review, Southeast Review, Ascent,* and *Turnrow.* Paul lives with his wife, Sally, and their children, Sarah, John, and Sam, in Durham, North Carolina.

Non Pro Nobis

John Bess

"Medic! Medic!"

The screams came from above me. I ran up the trail and into the woods. Red and white smoke billowed across the ground, obscuring everything. I spun around, searching for anything that looked like a patient. The wind shifted, causing a plume of smoke to spiral into the air, and I saw it. A boot in the dirt. I dove toward it, dropped my aid bag, and began evaluating the patient. The sound of machine guns ripped in the distance.

"Hey buddy, are you all right, are you OK?" I hollered. I quickly ran my hands from his head to his toe, looking and feeling for injuries.

A whistling scream pierced the sky. "Incoming!" a voice yelled in the distance. I leaned over my patient, creating a barrier between him and the metal fragments of the mortar round barreling toward us.

"No, no, no, goddamnit!" Sergeant First Class Genarro yelled as he stomped out of the woods in front of me. "You got to cover your patient, Bess." He shoved me down onto the practice dummy, forcing my face into the dirt. "You're a blanket, not an umbrella, son."

"Yes, sergeant, a blanket," I yelled.

Sergeant Genarro put his knee into my back and lowered his weight onto me. The air shot out of my lungs as the hard plastic of the mannequin pressed into my ribs.

"You got to cover him completely, Bess. You got to take that blast for your patient. Don't let him get another wound."

"Roger, sergeant." I tried to yell enthusiastically, but my lungs couldn't manage the effort.

"You feel that patient under your belly, private? You feel his bloody flesh in your face?"

"Yes, sergeant!"

"Is it uncomfortable?"

"Yes, sergeant!"

"Then you know you're doing it right." He leaned forward, pressing the mannequin deeper into my chest. "What's our motto, private?"

"Sergeant," I paused, trying to think. "*Non Pro Nobis . . . Non Pro Nobis Sed Aliis,* sergeant."

"And what does it mean, private?"

I thought about the lectures we received about the 105th Medical Regiment, the first formation of combat medics during the Mexican-American War, and the legacy and motto they had passed on to us.

"Not for ourselves but for others, sergeant!"

He grabbed me by the collar and yanked me to my feet. I didn't want to look at him, so I watched the last remnants of smoke from the grenades wreathe around his jungle boots and up his starched uniform. I knew what I'd see if I looked up: the Expert Field Medical Badge on his chest, the 1st Infantry Division combat patch on his shoulder, the disdain in his eyes.

"Don't you ever let your personal welfare come before your patient."

"I'm sorry, sergeant."

"Don't apologize to me, son. Apologize to the soldier you just killed," he said, giving the dummy a kick to the head.

I looked at the mannequin, dressed in fatigues and covered in fake blood. "Sorry."

"Medic. Hey medic, wake the fuck up."

I peeked out from my sleeping bag to see a red flashlight beam painting streaks across the inside of my track.

"Get up, private. We need you at Bulldog Two-One."

I rolled out of my bag fully dressed, slung on my LBE, and felt for my pistol and protective mask. Check. Grabbing my helmet in one hand and aid bag in the other, I lumbered out of my armored ambulance into the moonless black of another night in the South Korean countryside.

"What's wrong?" I asked the soldier walking briskly next to me.

"Don't know. That's your job, medic."

Medic. He practically spit the word at me. Here on the line, respect was reserved for the killers—tankers, scouts, and infantrymen. Back in the training battalion, seasoned medics like Sergeant Genarro had warned us that an unproven medic was about as welcome on the line as a case of heat rash. The only way to earn your keep, and the title "Doc," was by proving yourself, putting your patient's well-being ahead of your own.

I stumbled along, following the flashlight. I'd been in country exactly ten days, assigned to the 2-72 Armor Battalion for seven, and in the field with Bravo Company for three. This was my first duty assignment, and I was heading for my very first patient.

"Well, is he bleeding?" I asked.

"No, it's his stomach."

I ran through all the things I could remember from my training. Ruptured appendix, appendicitis, pancreatitis. Shit. I had no clue how to diagnose any of those things. I tried to remember which quadrant of the stomach held the pancreas. By the time we reached the tank, all I could remember was that the duodenum was in the upper right quadrant, but I had no idea what its function was or if it was even prone to causing pain. As I climbed up the side of the tank, two soldiers sitting on the back smoking cigarettes hollered toward the turret.

"You're fucked now, Hurley. They sent the private."

"Hey, Hurley, can I have your *Playboys* when you die?"

Inside the turret, a soldier sat doubled over in the commander's seat. Multicolored lights shone like a stained-glass window behind his head. Below him, in the belly of the tank, Sergeant Riley, whom I had met at the division's inprocessing station, sat reading a hot rod magazine. A small Walkman was wired into the tank's intercom system, reverberating Pearl Jam's "Evenflow" off the metallic walls.

I leaned into the turret and placed my hand on my patient's shoulder.

"Hey, buddy, how you doing?"

"Shit, not good," he said, turning his head slightly to look at me. "My stomach's fucking killing me."

"How long's it been going on?"

"Three days."

Well, I thought to myself, that rules out trauma.

"Can you point to where it hurts?"

He made a circular motion around his abdomen with his hand and said, "Everywhere."

Good, I thought, no point tenderness, probably something gastric.

"Can you lean back so I can feel?"

He tried to straighten himself in his seat, and I could tell that it made things worse.

"I don't want to come off the line," he said staring at his boots. "I can't go back to the rear."

My gut tightened. I squeezed his shoulder.

"Hey, that's why I'm here. Forward medicine, baby. I'll take care of you. Get you back in the shit."

I looked at Hurley, and my heart ached. At that moment I understood my mother's reason for leaving nursing. She used to always say she couldn't stand to see people suffer, that she cared about them too much to know she couldn't help them. I knew I had to do everything I could for him, so I focused on what I'd been taught.

I felt his abdomen with my left hand. No guarding, no rigidity. I asked a series of direct questions. He'd had worsening diarrhea since he'd been in the field. His head hurt. He was dizzy. He had no other symptoms.

"Can you come back to my track, so I can start an IV? You can rack out for a while, get some rest."

He looked at Sergeant Riley, who'd turned to see how he would respond.

"Can't you do it here?" Sure thing, I told him.

I started an IV and hung it from the whip antenna mounted to the turret.

"Look, you're dehydrated. You've been shitting out your electrolytes. I'm going to run this bag, then see how you're feeling." I pulled a bottle of Pepto from my aid bag and gave it to him. "Here, take a big drink of this every four hours starting now. Also, I don't want you eating the K–rats. That shit's too greasy. It'll run right through you. We need to keep some food and fluids in you for a day or two and see what happens. You guys have MREs?"

Sergeant Riley spoke up, "Just this box, four lunches for two days."

We had hot chow every morning and evening, K-rations, and ate the pre-packaged meals ready to eat for lunch. MREs are well known for causing constipation, which may be why the hot food was served so greasy, to even things out. But it wasn't working for my patient.

"I'll see if I can get more," I said.

I walked around our Area of Operations, searching for the mess trailer. Two cooks were getting breakfast ready, but they refused to give me a case of MREs. They had an entire pallet full, but no matter how hard I tried to explain the medical reason, they refused to give out a case to some private.

"If you can get authorization from the first sergeant," one of them said, "then we'll give them to you."

I walked to the Tactical Operations Center and found the soldier on radio watch. I explained the situation to him, but he said I'd have to come back in the morning, because he had strict orders not to disturb the first sergeant unless the North Koreans started a war.

I left the TOC and stood in the dark staring at nothing. What the hell was I supposed to do now? I headed for the mess trailer and snuck around back. I crouched low in the shadows, listening. The two cooks were joking and listening to rap music. The pallet full of MREs was only a few feet away. I thought about Corporal Hurley hunched over in pain. I thought about what would happen if I got caught: loss of rank, loss of pay, months of extra duty. Then I thought about the motto I had been forced to memorize: *Not for ourselves but for others.* I crawled forward, snatched two cases of MREs, and ran back to Bulldog Two-One.

The soldiers who'd been smoking were now stretched out on the back deck of the tank in their sleeping bags. I left the cases next to them and crawled up to check on Hurley. He was curled up in the cupola, his head propped on his helmet.

"How you feeling, troop?"

"Better, much better."

"Good." I took down the empty IV bag and removed the cannula from his arm. "Look, I had to swipe some MREs for you. There was no other way. Keep it between us."

Sergeant Riley shot me a hard look.

"Right, sergeant?"

He turned back to his magazine without a word.

"Stay away from those K-rations, corporal, and come see me tomorrow afternoon. OK?"

The next morning, before I was out of my sleeping bag, Sergeant Riley showed up at my track. He was carrying a tray of scrambled eggs, grits, toast, sausage, and two cartons of milk.

"Here you go, Doc," he said, setting the tray on the floor of my ambulance.

"What's this for?"

"For taking care of Hurley last night," he said, seeming surprised I would ask.

"How is he?"

"He's doing good. We're letting him sleep a bit. But he hasn't run off to the woods to shit once since you left."

"Good. That's good."

"You need anything else, Doc?"

I thought for a second about the things I could use at that moment—a hot shower, a cup of fresh coffee, a letter from home—then I pictured Hurley sleeping soundly for the first time in days.

"Nope, I think I've got everything I need. Thanks."

It was another quiet night in our little ER at Keller Army Community Hospital, the only twenty-four-hour facility at the United States Military Academy. Two of my medics were stretched out in the trauma room sleeping. The physician's assistant was upstairs in the call room, sleeping. And I was at the front desk, playing solitaire and surfing the Web for cheap apartments back home, some place to start my conversion back to civilian life after six years in uniform. I wanted to be sleeping, too. But I had to stay awake; somebody had to listen for the radio or be alert if a patient rolled in the door, and I was a staff sergeant, the second-highest-ranking NCO in the Emergency Room. It was my job to take care of my soldiers, to let them sleep. So I played another round of solitaire and thought about growing a beard when I got out.

"Keller base, State Patrol." The radio snapped to life next to my head. I jumped a little in my chair and took the call.

Flipping on the trauma room lights, I yelled, "We got a call!" as both medics hopped to their feet.

"What is it?" asked PFC Brice, a tall, lanky twenty-year-old.

"Unconscious male on the highway."

"Not Tommy Baldridge?" the other asked.

I looked at him, Sergeant Anthony Fischer, a solid medic and good NCO who'd just come to us from the 101st Airborne Division. "Don't know who it is, but we got the call."

Brice was already on his way out the door as I handed Fischer my notes from the call. "He's just outside Washington Gate, whoever it is."

"It better not be Baldridge," he said, putting on his hat and heading out into the dark morning. "I'll kick his fucking ass."

West Point sits on its own military reservation in New York. But part of that reservation, a stretch a little less than a mile long, crosses over State Road 218. We called it the Miracle Mile. If you got in a wreck anywhere in that stretch, our medics could respond and bring you straight to our ER, two minutes away. Wreck anywhere else and you had to wait for the volunteer services from Highland Falls to roll out of bed, get to the firehouse, then drive the fifteen minutes to come and get you.

Occasionally, a certain Thomas Baldridge would park his car on the shoulder of 218 and drink until he passed out. Eventually, the Rockland County sheriff's office or state police would find him, and because he'd claim some medical problem or another, they'd forget about taking him to the drunk tank and call us instead. He was a pleasant drunk, though. In fact, he liked coming to Keller.

I had just finished changing the bed paper in the trauma room when the ambulance rolled in. I decided not to wake the PA on duty. Mr. Baldridge was no drunker than usual, just complaining that his foot hurt. We had a pretty standard protocol for him: blood alcohol level, CBC, Chem 7, and IVs TKO.

Sergeant Fischer sat at the computer ordering the lab tests. "I don't see why we do all these tests. He doesn't have insurance. He can't pay for them."

"We can't refuse him service. His liver could be shot. He could have pneumonia. We'll check him out just to be sure."

I informed Mr. Baldridge we would be running some tests and that he'd feel a pinch. He lay placid as Brice drew his blood and started an IV.

"Hey, Tommy," Fischer hollered across the trauma room. "We're gonna put a tube in your dick so you don't piss all over our floor again."

"Use a condom cath," I said. There was no need to use an invasive and painful procedure on a simple drunk.

"Brice, put a condom cath on this guy," Fischer ordered.

"Why don't *you* do it?" Brice demanded. "I just drew his blood."

"That's 'Why don't you do it, *sergeant*?' And the answer is because I'm doing the paperwork. You've got penis duty, private. Enjoy."

Mr. Baldridge was moved to an exam room, where he promptly fell asleep. When the labs were sent off and the ambulance cleaned, Fischer and Brice resumed their naps in the trauma room. I stayed up, read the labs, changed the IV bag, and played more solitaire. Around five in the morning, Sergeant Fischer rolled out of bed.

"Did you take a look at homey's foot?"

I looked up from the computer. "Nope, totally forgot about it."

"Think we should? Just to make sure he doesn't have diabetes or something?"

"Yeah, sounds good."

Sergeant Fischer stepped into the exam room and turned on a small table lamp. I could hear him talking softly to Mr. Baldridge, but couldn't make out what he was saying. In a few minutes he returned.

"He's got an ingrown toenail. It's not infected yet, but it's getting there."

"You going to take it out?" I asked while I hunted for a red nine.

"Sure, might as well, or he'll just come back next week when he's spewing pus."

"Cool. Take Brice."

By the time the morning shift came in, Sergeant Fischer had walked Brice through the procedure. He was heading upstairs to grab breakfast from the hospital cafeteria as I finished up the chart note for the PA to sign when he woke up.

"I wonder what that would have cost him at St. Luke's," Fischer said, grabbing a handheld radio and turning it on.

"Probably five hundred bucks, easy," I said as I got up to join him.

"How much will we charge him?"

"Probably bill him two hundred at the most. Those toenail kits only cost us, like, eighteen dollars. Doesn't matter, he won't pay."

"You know that's why he comes here."

"Everyone knows it. But we can't deny him service."

"True, but we could have just sobered him up and ignored his foot."

"Where's the fun in that?" I asked as we climbed the stairs to the second floor.

"All I'm saying is that we always take it in the ass for this guy. Our hospital loses money every time we help him."

"It's not about us. You know that. *Non Pro Nobis*, right?"

"If you say so, sergeant."

After we paid for breakfast and were heading back downstairs, Sergeant Fischer stuck his head in the kitchen door and came out with a patient tray.

"Can't send the bastard home hungry," he said.

When I left the army, I struggled to find work in the medical field. Although the army had trained me in a slew of invasive procedures from chest tubes to venous cutdowns and given me the run of my own ER, the civilian world required licensing I didn't have just to change bedpans. Eventually, my experience reading lab reports got me a job at the Cardiac Care Center. It was the largest cardiology practice in the state, with eighteen physicians and satellite clinics in seven different towns. They even had their own heart hospital with state-of-the-art diagnostic facilities.

I ran the lipid clinic—ordering, reading, and reporting lab values for our patients' cholesterol levels and managing their prescriptions. One winter morning, I was leaning back in my office chair with the phone to my ear, staring at the ceiling.

"No, I'm sorry, Mrs. Segura, I haven't heard back from Dr. Roberts yet. He's been in surgery all week and has only been able to come by the office on his lunch breaks." I waited, listening. "No, ma'am, your husband's LDL is fine. It's his HDL, the good cholesterol, I'm worried about. That's why I asked Dr. Roberts to change his medication."

I leaned toward the computer screen, checking my e-mail account, as she read off her husband's medications.

"I don't want Mr. Segura to run out of medication either," I replied. "Tell you what, I'll leave you a month's supply of Lescol at the front desk. When I get your husband's chart back from Dr. Roberts, I'll call in the new prescription to your pharmacy, OK?"

I opened Mr. Segura's history in my lipid management database. He'd been on the same cholesterol meds for years. Lescol was one of the older statins on the market and wasn't as effective in raising HDL as others. This wasn't an isolated incident, and Lescol wasn't the only drug. I routinely received orders from a handful of our physicians that didn't fit current best practice. They could be counted on to order specific drugs almost regardless of the patient's particulars.

Dr. Roberts's small office was overflowing with papers and charts. A half-eaten chicken sandwich and fries sat on the corner of his desk. The wilted, brown lettuce told me it had been there for a few days. Dr. Roberts was leaning over his desk, talking on the phone, and taking sips from his "I'd Rather Be Fishing" coffee cup. I waited, staring at the row of snapshots taped to the bookshelf above his desk. A few pictures of his twin daughters. A shot of him in front of a mountain stream, decked out in hip waders, flannel shirt, and scruffy beard, holding a large fish. On his head was a beat-up Novartis ballcap. Next to this was a Post-it note written on Novartis stationery. A bold, flowery hand had written, "Dr. Rob—How was Canada? Hope you enjoyed the trip. Vicki."

I knew Vicki. She was the Novartis pharmaceutical rep, one of the many from various companies who were always hanging around the office chatting up the docs.

When Dr. Roberts hung up the phone, I walked up to him and said good morning.

"Oh, hey, John," he said. His rusty hair was matted to his head, and the wrinkled scrubs peeking through his crisp lab coat told me he'd been in the cath lab all night. I tried to minimize the typical ex-military, too-much-coffee, let's-get-it-done tone of my voice.

"Do you happen to have Johnny Segura's chart?"

He looked through the piles on his desk and pulled it out. There on the top were the prescriptions I had written. It was common practice for techs to write out prescriptions so all the doctors had to do was sign if they agreed. I had provided Dr. Roberts the two top therapeutic choices for Mr. Segura's condition. Above them was my own hand-written Post-it note in the cryptic shorthand of our practice.

Dr. Rob—

HDL<39, LDL 88 on current Rx. Δ to Tricor 160 mg qd? Lipitor/ Niaspan?

—John

Dr. Roberts looked at the recent lipid test clipped to the chart, then scrawled the following prescription change next to it: Gemfib 600/Lescol 40 bid.

"Here you go," he said, handing me the file and tossing my prescriptions in the shredder.

I read his note and held a finger up as if I could stop time for a moment while I thought about his decision. "Do you really think this is the best choice?"

"Yep."

"But numerous studies have shown Tricor to be the most effective course of treatment for ACH patients with low HDL."

"Really?" he said. He spun in his chair to face me. "Remind me again which medical school you went to?"

"Never mind," I said. "Lescol it is."

I walked to the storeroom, seething. I couldn't help feeling we were screwing Mr. Segura over by not giving him the best meds possible. I began filling a plastic bag with sample packs of Lescol and pamphlets on managing cholesterol. I pulled a pen and blue Post-it pad out of my lab coat, scribbled Mr. Segura's name, and placed it on the distorted CCC logo emblazoned across the bulging package. As I was putting the pad back in my pocket, I noticed the large Tambocor (3M) logo across the top. Every writing utensil, magnet, and day planner in our office was from some pharmaceutical company or another. It was just part of working in a civilian medical practice, so much so I never thought much about it. I realized that in the army we gave the cheapest, most effective drug available, generic if possible. The docs at CCC rarely prescribed generics.

I opened Mr. Segura's bag and cocked my head to read the side of a Lescol box. Manufactured by Novartis. My cheek twitched. I felt my jaw tighten. I finally understood: Not for others but for ourselves.

I'd like to tell you that I marched upstairs and filed a complaint, that I exposed this travesty to the world. But I did nothing. I knew a patient's health was being compromised for some grand fishing expedition, yet I did nothing. To this day I'm not exactly sure why. I had gone into the medical field to help people, and I felt like I was making a difference. But at that moment, I learned medicine was not inherently about helping others. For the first time, I saw the medical field from the practice's perspective, from the perspective of pharmaceutical companies and others for whom it was a moneymaking opportunity. Maybe I'd been idealistic. Maybe I'd been naive. But now I was just disillusioned. Worse, by not saying anything, I was complicit. My silence may have harmed Mr. Segura. It surely didn't help. I made the decision to just do my job—answer the phones, fill prescriptions—and something inside me, some bit of the great pride I felt as a caretaker of my fellow man, vanished.

Six months later, the entire nursing staff was gathered in the Cardiac Care Center's conference room. We were seated around a huge, oval table facing a bounty of coffee and doughnuts. We were all there but one: Maggie Shea, our senior nurse. She'd been let go the week before. The rest of the nursing office, we were told, would take up her duties. We would do more with less.

This was the mantra of Mike Spinogle, the fellow aiming a laser pointer at the screen in front of us. Several smaller cardiology practices in the region had merged and were literally giving us a run for our money. So the partners had brought Mike in from some big East Coast practice to make us more profitable.

It was his idea to fire Maggie. It was also his idea to stop our free prescriptions for indigenous patients. My office mate, Tom Keeley, who ran the indigenous patient program, was promptly let go as well. Everyone in the nursing office wondered who was next. People were dusting off their résumés and preparing arguments for their own necessity within the Cardiac Care Center. It was this tense bunch that sat before Mike eating doughnuts and drinking coffee, because that's what you do when you're a team player. You eat the doughnuts. You drink the coffee. And you keep your mouth shut.

Mike was striding back and forth in front of the screen. He reminded me of George C. Scott in the intro to *Patton*, except Mike had Italian leather loafers instead of jackboots, a laser pointer instead of a riding crop.

"Everyone gets the tunnel," he said, referring to the imaging tunnel of the CT scan. "We've got studies upon studies that allow us to order MRIs or CTs on every patient. Congenital heart disease?" he paused for effect and turned on his heel. "MRI." He looked at me and pointed, "High lipids?"

"CT angiograph?"

"Bingo!" He snapped his hand back and pumped his fist. "Nurses, if you think someone needs an echocardiogram, order a function MRI." He hit a button on his laptop, and his PowerPoint screen changed to show a list of prices. "Insurance only pays \$178 for an echo, but they'll give us \$312 for an MRI. So we're phasing out our echo lab. We're going to create two new exam rooms to increase our patient flow. An extra hundred patients a month will allow us to generate unprecedented revenue for the practice."

I left the meeting feeling like I'd just been subjected to a fast-food training film. Would you like an angiogram with your coronary artery disease? Supersize that EKG?

I retreated to my office and listened to my voicemails. Half of them were for Tom. The operators didn't know what to do with the frustrated patients now that Tom and his program were gone, so they were sending them to me. I wrote down the names and phone numbers and began calling them back. The first number I dialed was for an elderly patient living on the Navajo reservation. I held my breath while the phone rang and sighed deeply when her answering machine picked up.

"Hello, Mrs. Yazzie? This is John Bess from the Cardiac Care Center returning your call." Mike was passing by my office and stopped in my doorway. He leaned on my doorjamb, waiting. "In regards to the free medications you were receiving, I'm sorry to inform you that our practice will no longer be offering that service. You can apply for help directly from the manufacturers, and if you'd like, I can help you get those forms filled out."

Mike leaned in over my monitor, whispering. "Don't forget the CT."

"I'd also like to tell you that we are now offering cardiac imaging, both CT and MRI, exclusively to our patients. Feel free to call us if you'd like to set up an appointment."

Mike gave me a thumbs-up and a healthy nod as I hung up the phone. "Good work. Hey, I heard you had some extra room in here," he said looking around my office. "Yeah, this will do. We're going to move you over to the records room, set you up a phone and computer there. We can get another exam room in here, increase our flow. How's that sound?"

"Sounds great, Mike."

I wanted to tell him what it really sounded like—one more plan to shaft the patients in order to make a buck. I wanted to tell him how I had come to despise the health care system. I wanted to tell him that I couldn't look myself in the eye anymore. But I knew my words were pointless. There was money to be made, and somewhere along the line, some people would be helped. But some would be lied to. Some would die. All I could do was make sure it was never again a result of something I did, or, as in Johnny Segura's case, failed to do.

As Mike walked away, I picked up my stethoscope and left my office. I wandered around the building for a while. I slowly headed toward the administrative offices. No one was around, and all the doors were locked. I pulled out my heart-shaped Plavix Post-its, scribbled a letter of resignation, and slapped it on the Human Resources door. I packed up my office and, without fanfare or explanation, walked away from medicine for good.

John D. Bess received his MFA from the University of New Mexico, where he still teaches various writing courses. He is finishing his first book, an essay cycle about his tumultuous relationship with his father, titled *Still Life with Guns,* and researching his second, a historical novel about the Colfax County War. He lives in Albuquerque with his son, Jacob, two German shepherds, and a vast array of guitars.

Saving My Breath

Tamara Dean

On the Sunday night after my overdose, when I was certain no one would be there to answer, I called my internist's office. I styled my voice to sound casual and perky, evoking a 1950s receptionist. "Just to let you know, I had a seizure." I told him I was taking myself off the medications he'd recently prescribed, the combination that had caused the overdose, then hung up.

Dr. T. and his nurses phoned my home and office every day for the next week, leaving messages that increased in their urgency but varied little in their content: "Call our office immediately." *Lawsuit* was the unspoken subtext. The tone, however, was commanding, as if I were the impossible patient and he the earnest doc. I doodled on a nearby memo pad, satisfied, while I listened to these daily messages. I would wait, and make them wait. I would talk to them when I pleased, calmly and confidently. I'd been a dutiful patient too long.

My lungs had troubled me since birth, wheezing to slow me down or seizing up to send me to the emergency room. When I was an adolescent, adult doses of certain bronchodilators had left me anxious and paranoid. For a year I was convinced I had lice. I would scrape my scalp, pull out my hair strand by strand for examination, and compel my mother to check me repeatedly, even waking her in the night to do so. After one emergency room visit and a fresh batch of prescriptions, I began to hallucinate. Worms corkscrewed out of my flesh, walls melted, and just beyond my reach, purple and pink spots squirmed like paramecia under a microscope. No one then—or ever—had suggested I should stop taking a prescribed medicine, and I hadn't.

But as a recent college graduate with my first unshared apartment and a real job, I was alone in dealing with medical professionals. As if the seizure had shaken me out of a mute complacency about my condition, I decided to begin defying doctors. It seemed a fresh, original idea. It would also take practice.

Dr. T. was my father's age. He was all but bald, he mumbled, and he loved golf. On the bookshelf behind his desk sat a photograph of his daughter, taken in the mid-seventies. She wore thick, plastic-rimmed glasses and a necklace dangling a gold heart, nearly the same glasses and necklace that appeared in my own fourth-grade picture. Nearby was a recent photo of her grown up; now she sported the same hairstyle as mine and wore the same type of soft sweater.

Though harried, Dr. T. always fit me in on short notice, like the day, six weeks before the seizure, when I realized I was in trouble. Blue-tinged fingernails didn't strike me as odd, but I was alarmed when I couldn't walk the ten steps from bed to bathroom in my efficiency apartment without gasping and stopping to catch my breath. Chronic asthmatics adjust to lower oxygen levels, to sipping and conserving air—don't laugh, don't shout, don't sing, don't run. And herein lies the conundrum of speaking up: is saving your breath self-censorship or self-preservation? Often I remained silent not because I felt acquiescent or content but because the matter wasn't important enough to warrant the necessary expense of oxygen and the heaving of lungs and diaphragm. On a "worth the breath" scale, for example, complaining about a mistaken order at a restaurant was a zero, as was asking doctors follow-up questions. But I couldn't tell what marked the upper bound. What could possibly justify the effort of angry rebuttal?

I shuffled the three blocks between my office and Dr. T.'s, staying close to the buildings, pausing to lean against the concrete. The nurse took blood from the artery in my wrist and then analyzed its oxygen saturation. Normal adults experience nearly 99 percent saturation, while asthmatics are often closer to 90 percent. Mine was 54. Or this is what I remember Dr. T. telling me as he flashed the printout, which resembled a dime-store receipt, so I could see the numbers for myself.

"I'm calling an ambulance," he said.

I followed his orders, and was confined for a week, because of overcrowding, to a room in the terminal ward with moaning, deeply suffering patients. (A doctor on evening rotations told me cheerfully, "You're my only non-AIDS patient.") When I was released, jubilant to be free, I was taking more than my usual multiple medications, jotting dosage times and amounts on the backs of envelopes, carrying loose capsules in my coat and jeans pockets, and occasionally forgetting what I last took and when. Disorganized perhaps, but still dutiful.

A month afterward, on Saint Patrick's Day, 1990, I was visiting friends in Chicago, the city all new to me—the green river, the parade with the mayor in a Leprechaun's hat, waving, police lining the route on a cool, damp Saturday. My friends were drunk and determined to get drunker, so we walked to a bar and ordered a round. When they wandered off to cruise the dark corners, I quickly abandoned my rum and its chemical taste. I felt queasy and irritable; I couldn't trust my senses. A young man next to me struck up a conversation. All I remember of him is the jet-fuel stench of his leather jacket, though this might have been my brain's creation. Had I felt better I might have taunted the boy with something feminist and tough, but instead I barely spoke, barely looked him in the eye.

Then began the strange dance. My head snapped to the right, to the right, to the right. "Oh God," I tried to say, and I was aware of my mouth opening for the "Oh," but likely nothing came out. Next my right arm also took up flailing, to the right, to the right. No force to stop it, within or without. I was as much surprised as frightened. I didn't know my body could move so wildly without my consent. I felt no pain, just the opposite—a powerless relaxation, as if in freefall—and registered that this was remarkable. Then my body began lurching, forward and back, forward and back, a ball being tossed between giants. Forward, back—that's the last I remembered.

I've constructed an image of myself on the floor in my black coat, continuing the seizure without consciousness, people moving aside to give me room and yelling for the bartender and my friends. One friend leapt, she later told me, to where I lay. She also said, "Don't ever do that again," but there ended our discussion about the incident, and I never asked. I didn't want to own the image of a sick person—an asthmatic, especially. Asthma is the nuisance of the fat kid on the playground. As an adult I rarely mentioned it outside of doctors' offices.

Next I heard sirens and thought, blandly, *a city, someone's been hurt.* Then the all-white interior of an ambulance materialized.

"What's going on?" I asked.

"You lost consciousness. We're not sure what happened."

"Where am I?"

"You're in Chicago."

"No I'm not. I live in Washington."

"What's your name?"

"I know my name," I said with disgust.

"Who's the president?"

"Don't—" *be ridiculous, you mean they really ask who's president?* I lacked the energy to say more.

An IV had been put in my arm. One of my friends sat facing me beyond the end of the stretcher. I smelled her cloud of alcohol and wanted to insist to the paramedics that I hadn't drunk anything myself, but then I blanked out again.

I regained consciousness in the emergency room. My friends stood inside the thin curtain next to my bed.

"We need you to take your pants off," a nurse said.

"Why?"

"To take your temperature."

But no one does that anymore, I thought, and then did it anyway, uncomplaining. I was accustomed to following the orders of medical professionals.

Lying on the narrow cot, I still couldn't remember traveling to Chicago, nor the beginning of the seizure, but facts pointed to my not being at home in suburban Washington, D.C. If I kept quiet, I thought, I might fool them, or my memory might seep back.

Or had I already spoken? Without my knowledge, the emergency room professionals had assessed my condition—they'd taken blood, known I wasn't drunk, and determined the cause for my seizure. My body had communicated in lieu of my brain.

"Your theophylline level was twenty-eight," a man said in a hasty and resigned tone, as if he saw these cases every day, as if theophylline was being dealt on the seediest corners of the city, right after heroin.

Theophylline, a chemical that occurs naturally in chocolate, tea, and coffee, causes the bronchial muscles to relax. In concentrated pill form it has enjoyed popularity as an asthma treatment, though not recently. It's one of those tricky meds that's effective and nonlethal only within a certain range. Levels over twenty milligrams per liter in the blood cause adverse reactions—from nausea, anxiety, and tachycardia to seizures and even death. Theophylline levels can be augmented by other substances, including ciproflaxin. When I was in the hospital back home, my doctor had prescribed ciproflaxin as a precaution against bronchial infection. It was a new antibiotic then, but its interactions were well known. I shouldn't have been taking both drugs.

I was aware that medical treatments could go awry, but only in a theoretical sense, in the same way I knew that a person could drown in a bathtub. It *rarely* happened, and it certainly wouldn't happen to me. But, in fact, a report released in July 2006 by the Institute of Medicine concluded that 7,000 people die each year in the United States as a result of errors in prescribing medication. Things could have gone much worse for me. Still, until the seizure I had not imagined that a doctor I knew, a doctor writing my prescriptions, might prove patently wrong.

"You could be a millionaire," a pharmaceutical company executive told me. "Sue the doctor. It's a slam-dunk."

But I didn't want a court battle. I wanted to take charge of my health, even if I wasn't sure what that meant or how to achieve it. I began with defiance; *that* would be worth my breath.

Doctors call it noncompliance, and understandably, it vexes them. Willfully or ignorantly, patients neglect to take their medicine, miss appointments, ignore their diets, keep smoking, forgo physical therapy, or never follow up on requested tests. By some current estimates half of all Americans treated for any illness or condition don't take their prescribed medications properly, and half of all American asthma patients are, in general, noncompliant. In fact, noncompliance has reached such epidemic proportions that some health professionals propose making it a medical diagnosis, a disease in its own right. An industry of educational tools, researchers, and consultants has coalesced around the challenge of getting patients to conform to doctors' orders. But in my case, the notion of noncompliance was empowering. I would no longer quietly obey the experts. After all, they had proven they weren't experts.

• • •

In the two days following the seizure, I slept greedily and deeply, and afterward, as if my brain had been plugged into a charger, I could piece together memories of the period I'd lost, beginning with my flight to Chicago. I recalled my seatmate, a nurse, saying she could tell from one look that I was taking corticosteroids. I recalled the parade, the bar, the beginning of the seizure, the emergency room. By the time I returned home I'd regained as much knowledge as I will ever have about that weekend, and that night I called Dr. T. to leave my message.

Eventually, we met. I expected a debriefing in which he would express regrets and I would question him about the best course of treatment going forward. But he never admitted that the Chicago emergency room's diagnosis was valid. Instead he admonished me, claiming that the seizure might indicate something more serious: epilepsy, a brain tumor.

"Oh, come on," I said.

"We can't rule it out. This is very unusual, and very serious. Do you understand?" He prescribed antiseizure medication and referred me to a neurologist, a friend of his.

The neurologist was haughty and young and his waiting-room reading material consisted of nothing but medical journals, which were unintelligible. The art was Miró reproductions, poorly framed. After the first office visit, during which he questioned me and performed a number of simple tests, he recommended an EEG. When that came back fine, he prescribed a sleep-deprived EEG. When that came back fine, he prescribed an MRI.

I earned $13,500 per year in a job with the federal government. My health insurance paid 80 percent of medical expenses, but the remaining 20 percent of my hospital and doctor bills that year, before the seizure, had purged my savings, and new charges remained unpaid. My share of an MRI would cost hundreds of dollars.

"No," I said. "I can't afford it. And I don't need it."

Some alternative healers call asthma the disease of self-suffocation, a manifestation of the inability or unwillingness to express oneself, to speak up. I had never thought that was my problem (wasn't I merely saving my breath out of self-preservation?), but then, I was shaking as I contradicted this neurologist.

He looked up from his desk, brow lifted. He stared for a moment. "What state do you live in?"

"Maryland."

"You've had a seizure. Legally, I could have your driver's license taken away."

I stared back.

"What if you were driving a car when you had that seizure?" he demanded. "What if you were driving a car and hit another car? Huh? And what if, in that other car, there was a little baby? And what if you killed that little baby when you hit that car? Then what?"

I tell myself now that had I not felt so ill and weak, I would have laughed at his histrionics and walked out right then. But the truth is I can still picture that imaginary car (a gray sedan), the curved section of road just north of my apartment, woods thick on either side, where the accident would occur, and the way the cars would strike and crumple on impact. I still picture the baby seat (navy blue, upholstered) too, though curiously, the seat has always been empty.

In a 1987 study published in *Social Science Medicine*, researcher Irena Heszen-Klemens wrote that in taped conversations between physicians and noncompliant patients, physicians relied most frequently on "authoritarian tactics" and "medical threats [to convey] the doctor's point in an indulgent atmosphere." She also found that not only were these tactics ineffective but they actually reduced patient compliance. Yet in her study groups, she concluded, the doctors' "ego-defensive tactics predominated." In a similar study from that time, doctors questioned admitted that at least 50 percent of the time they relied on authoritarian tactics to urge compliance.

Cooperative, concordant, coordinating, cohealing. These words have been suggested to replace "compliant," which was introduced into the medical lexicon in the 1970s. Perhaps because of research such as Ms. Heszen-Klemens's, doctors are now educated in ways of gaining a patient's trust, like honoring needs and lifestyles, taking time to answer questions, and explaining why a treatment is well advised. All of which seems like plain common sense.

I did have the MRI, though I was in tears when I left the neurologist's office, hating the doctor and agonizing over the cost. Results from the test showed nothing abnormal. Dr. T. never mentioned the seizure again. I stopped taking the antiseizure medication, just as I stopped taking the antiheartburn medication I'd required because of the antiseizure medication, without asking permission or telling him what I'd done.

As a former engineer raised in a household of sensible scientists, I have never believed in ghosts, apparitions, spirit guides, or voices that announce themselves sans human form. If someone told me he heard or saw anything of that sort, I would dismiss his experience as fantasy. Even if *I* heard or saw such a thing, I would dismiss it. Which is exactly what I had done when I heard the voice. Probably, I thought, it was the drugs—or a lack of oxygen.

Nearly three months before the seizure, I was spending Christmas vacation at my parents' house. My medications at the time—steroids, multiple bronchodilators, antihistamines, even a narcotic painkiller—had left me shaking yet stupefied, exhausted yet unable to sleep. In the middle of the night I drew a bath, then abandoned it after a minute's soaking to pace the hallway, still wet, a white towel draped over my shoulders.

My mother woke and asked, "What's wrong?"

I shook my head. "I'm dead to the world."

Later, lying in bed, I wondered how to get back, to live. I'd been considering a change of environment. I lived in a mildewed basement apartment with old carpeting. My only window faced the pavement level of a parking lot where neighbors kept their cars running to warm them each morning, the tailpipes pointed my way. And the air in Washington was muggy, always pressing down, choking.

I might or might not have been falling asleep.

"Just go to Madison."

Audible, deliberate, and calm. Distinctly a voice, without a human presence. In the room with me. Never before and never since have I heard such a thing.

But Madison? Wisconsin? I'd never been there, didn't know anyone there, had no job prospects there. Although I had nothing against the place, I also didn't have any reason to move to Madison. I dismissed the idea, along with the very idea of a voice, and returned to D.C. at the end of December.

But after the seizure, after my first attempts at contradicting doctors, I remembered this voice, which of course, I'd never actually forgotten. I had little to lose. I quit my job and moved to Madison.

Speaking up, surviving. Both drew on and generated more self-empowerment, just as they drew on and generated more breath. My attempts before the move were timid beginnings, but now I was committed to healing myself. I just had to figure out how.

Any sufferer of chronic illness will attest that every acquaintance and stranger knows a surefire cure for her ailment. And no matter how crazy the cures sound, if there is a remote chance they'll work, she will try them. Over the years I had experimented with chiropractic manipulation, creative visualization, acupuncture, massage therapy, hypnosis, homeopathic medicines, herbs, tinctures, teas, and special diets—all without positive results, and in some cases to the further detriment of my health. People on planes especially love to give advice. One copassenger said her son was completely cured from asthma through rigorous exercise. "You must exercise. Try running." she said.

I nodded amiably.

Nor was moving to a different city a magical cure, of course. In Madison I still needed prescriptions. Breathing, I wrote in my journal of that time, felt like trying to row out of a vortex with my ribs as oars. Doctors tell us that with this disease, *exhalation* is the difficult part—the wheezing, constricted half of respiration. But experience told me in-breath and out-breath were equal struggles.

Luck brought me to Dr. O., an allergy specialist and renowned expert on indoor air quality and its effects on breathing. He was short and myopic, wistful when lauding Tommy Dorsey and goofy when he hustled between examining rooms. Upon meeting me he said, "I don't know what you do, but you're hired. What a handshake!"

Dr. O. made no assumptions. He evaluated my allergy tests, family history, lung capacity tests, and chest X-rays, which revealed that my ribcage had stretched outward from so many years of the rowing, the fighting for air. He asked if my house had carpeting, a basement, pets, or mold—all potential allergen sources. He loaned me his favorite textbooks, their pages bookmarked and dog-eared, to take home. "Here, read this bit about eosinophils and leukotrienes," he advised after giving a brief tutorial on the molecules that contributed to bronchoconstriction.

Then he said, "So. What do you think is causing the problem?"

"Uhhh." I stalled. Here was my invitation to speak up, and yet I was dumbfounded by his question, by the very fact that a doctor had asked my opinion.

It wasn't that I hadn't scrutinized my breathing every day, tried to correlate difficulties with particular environments, stressors, foods, exercise, or laughing fits, but that I couldn't detect any causal relationships. Asthma had become the impossible, mercurial roommate whom it's easier to avoid than try to analyze or appease.

"I have no idea. It never gets better, so how do I know what makes it worse?"

He nodded sagely, and I felt like I'd blown my chance. Again. Despite my resolve. Thankfully, though, he left the question open for me to return to, and I did.

During the next ten years I grew comfortable telling him not only what I thought was affecting my breathing but also why I mistrusted doctors, which medications didn't work, when I would stop taking a drug, and why I questioned new prescriptions. He respected me, listened, summarized the latest research, and urged me to try new therapies. My asthma was present, but well managed. I could walk—exercise, even—and my fingernails were rarely blue. Even better, perhaps, I'd progressed from unstudied defiance to an assured, *concordant* partnership with my doctor to save my breathing.

Then, in September 2002, on a trip to Europe, I forgot to take my three daily medicines. But unlike with past slipups, my breathing didn't seem to suffer, neither in the subsequent hours nor the next day. Emboldened, I abandoned the prescriptions in my suitcase for the rest of the ten-day trip and then for weeks after I returned home. I was mysteriously fine.

For the following three years I forgot about my medications—and asthma. I felt not just well but exuberantly healthy. Energetic and collected. Liberated. Quite literally, I was given a breather. Or had I *taken* it? Had the remission been a fluke, or had greater involvement in my own health care caused it to happen? I wasn't sure.

Six months before the trip to Europe, I'd moved to a new place with no carpeting or basement. I'd also adopted two new pursuits: breathing meditation and exercising with a trainer, pushing myself to an extreme at the gym, running when I could and lifting weights. One bit of recent asthma research suggests that chronic inflammation can alter the physiology of bronchial tubes, making them more constricted and sensitive ever after. If they're malleable, does it also follow that they could be expanded? Might I have stretched and made my bronchi less sensitive through the hard breathing of exercise?

I suspect my relief was due to a combination of effort and environment, but I've learned that cures don't come simply, swiftly, or even logically, and that despite our desire for definitive fixes, we must remain open to mystery.

Last year I moved to a tiny, rural town, where my habits of meditation and vigorous exercise gave way to a life overscheduled with new responsibilities and where I, reluctantly, rented a place with carpet and a basement. The asthma, my old ghost, my closest, constant companion, resurfaced. After a December week of sleepless nights and dizzy-headed days, I called a coworker whose husband is one of the few doctors in town. She gave me the other doctors' numbers but said about her husband, "You know, two of our kids have bad asthma, so he's very experienced with it, personally as well as professionally."

I liked him, but when he tried to give advice or help diagnose me I felt like an addict simply there for my fix.

"Yeah, I know," I said, cutting him off as he began to explain how chronic asthmatics adjust to lower oxygen levels.

I only wanted the prescriptions, and I planned to take medication only as long as necessary until I could get back into my good habits, when the disease would surely retreat.

But my friend's husband recognized a noncompliant. As he wrote four prescriptions he gazed at me shrewdly and said, "If you skip any medications don't let it be the inhaled steroid. That'll do you the most good." And once again before I left the examination room: "Remember, if you decide to not fill all these prescriptions, make sure you at least fill this one."

Speaking up in the interest of my health, it seemed, required being honest with him. I had told him about my history, and now I added that most likely I would fill only the inhaled steroid prescription. He nodded.

Asthma treatments have progressed dramatically in the sixteen years since my seizure. Theophylline is rarely prescribed. Inhaled steroids have become common, and their limited scope of side effects is a big improvement over that of the oral steroids I took for the better part of twenty years. Indeed, the inhaled steroid is the only medication I've used, and I use it sporadically. Many weeks pass when my breathing is perfect. Only occasionally does it get difficult, and never to the extreme that it did in my twenties. I realize the risks of my choice: the inhaled steroid is not fast-acting, but preventative and most effective if taken daily. Still, I'm content with my decision and my breathing.

Last week I went to our local drugstore to pick up a refill. The older ladies behind the pharmacy desk dawdled and giggled inexplicably. They happened to be laughing with each other as they answered the phone, they laughed when I gave them my prescription number and chuckled to themselves when they couldn't find my bag in the plastic tub behind the counter. But when the clerk rang up the inhaled steroid refill she looked grim.

"Two hundred fifty-eight dollars. Oh my."

"My insurance doesn't cover it," I shrugged.

"That's terrible."

She was required to call over the pharmacist—a stately, older man—to complete the transaction. He glanced at a sticker on the little white bag and then at me.

"You're not taking it enough," he said sternly. "You haven't refilled this in three months. You are to use this twice a day and refill it each month."

Two thoughts arose in quick succession. First: "*You paternalistic bastard, how dare you profess to know better than I do what my body needs!*" and the second, which I voiced confidently while smiling: "Oh, I have a stockpile of samples from the doctor."

The pharmacist eyed me. "OK, then."

"At that price, you almost have to," the clerk said, and together we laughed.

Tamara Dean earned her MFA in Fiction Writing from Vermont College
and writes fiction, essays, and technical books. Her creative nonfiction has recently appeared
in *Orion*, *Sustainable Eating*, and *Spring Wind*. Her book *The Human-Powered Home*
will be published in 2008 by New Society Publishers.

Watching My Mother Hallucinate

Diana Hume George

"You look so much like your mom," says the starched, very pregnant nurse at the rehab unit where Mom has been sent to recover from her hip surgery, "only younger."

My pulse skips whenever someone says this. The first half of my life was devoted to being nothing like her. I thought we were not members of the same species, never mind the same family. Even now, decades later, when I feel close to her and am her primary emotional support, even now, when I have reclaimed her last name as part of my own, even now, when I no longer twitch after an hour in her presence, and do not bolt for the door as soon as I can, but stay as long as I am able, still the idea that our relationship shows on our faces makes me uncomfortable. When I hear her tones in my own voice, I want to take back whatever I said, for it will surely have been admonitory ("Be careful") or blaming ("If you hadn't done that—") or authoritative ("I know all about it") or high-handed ("You listen to me, mister-man"). It happens when I am tired and witless, and lately that's a lot.

Which is when I am likeliest to slip in other ways. I felt scared and sad a few years ago when Mom first called me her mother instead of her daughter. "This," she said with a grand introductory hand gesture involving the wrist, "is my mother, Alice Ruth." That time, after saying hello to the health care worker and exchanging a secret look with her, I excused myself, went into the bathroom, and sat down on the toilet seat to have the briefest possible identity crisis. Mom was losing her grip, and I'd known it, but there's nothing quite like that first time the role-reversal comes out of a parent's mouth. It rips you up.

Now, though, I'm used to it, or I think I am. Reminded of how much I look like her (only younger), I extend my hand to introduce myself to the new doctor at this rehab center. "Hello," I say, my grasp firm and in control of this institutional situation, "Janice is my daughter." But I do not know that I have said this. It simply slipped out. He and the nurse glance at each other, then laugh. I hear the echo of my words and emit a mirthless chirp, do my best Gilda Radner eye roll, excuse myself, go into the bathroom, and kick the toilet. Too tired to choke up. I'll do that later while I'm driving home from this place that I've left her, where I promised I'd never leave her, this rehab unit of a nursing home, to the residential wing of which I shall consign her permanently next week.

She's my daughter, all right. I'm her mother, all right. And like her when the situations were reversed, I make arbitrary decisions to control and tame her, to confine and isolate her, to make her life miserable for no good reason, or so it must seem to her. She feels I am against her, even though I explain that it's all for the best. Where have I heard that one before? I dust off the worn phrases she threw at me and I throw them back, moldy and lame. "This has to be done. It's for your own good."

The circle is unbroken, by and by, Lord, by and by. I watch her like she used to watch me. I keep a zealous eye on her meds in particular. Last year I copy-edited a book on the overmedication of the nation's elderly. Seventeen meds is typical, one prescribed for the side effects created by another, created by another. That would never happen to *my* mom, not while *I* am in charge. (Even in this, I see her high hand upon my personality in my illusion of control.)

She'd been on only one med for the previous two years, a mild dose of an antidepressant. One time we upped it to see if it might affect her obsessive use of the emergency call button at her assisted living facility—up to twenty times a day she demands attention, wants the curtain open, no, shut, the window open, no, closed, the clock angle changed, the Chapstick located, the bottle of alcohol removed from the table occupied by the radio for fear of spontaneous combustion, the leftover milk shake disposed of because it undoubtedly has a high bacterial count from the hour it's been unrefrigerated, the water level checked on her humidifier. The water is always at the same level, but that does not matter, she must have it checked to prevent fire. That window matter is crucial, for what if a deer jumped through the window (it is open three inches) into her room, perhaps biting her and spreading rabies? But when the increased dosage made no difference and caused her discomfort, I had it cut back. I mean to say, I am on top of this meds thing. Calcium, Tylenol for arthritis, an anti-inflammatory when her system can deal with it, mild laxatives when needed. No big bad pills with columns of side effects. I will not permit it. Or wouldn't if I knew about it. But the medical people don't always tell you what they're doing.

Here's what happened. When she fell down and was hospitalized needing X-rays and tests, my control over her medications dissolved. I didn't know that the moment you enter a hospital, all bets are off and any meds the doctors order are on. Nothing was broken that time, but they decided to do other tests it would have been irresponsible of me to disallow. They also evaluated her psychologically and found her "mildly paranoid." When I inquired as to how that diagnosis was reached, it emerged that they'd asked her if she ever felt people were against her, and she'd answered "Yes, sometimes." How to tell them that this isn't paranoia, it's reality, because Mom's an impossibly demanding person? Some of the aides *are* "against" her, with good reason—at minimum wage, perhaps her correction of their grammar is not welcome. "Don't say *I seen*, say *I saw*," she instructs them, and refuses to sign paperwork if it contains a misspelled word. "Write it over again," she demands, "and then *perhaps* I shall sign it."

Because of that diagnosis, one of her doctors ordered three psychoactive meds, and upped the dosages daily without informing me. Mom would take anything given to her by a man in a white coat—and it would have to be a man, because like many women in her generation, she does not trust women. On these new medications, she became truly paranoid. Moved from the hospital to rehab for her merely bruised hip, she became convinced she'd been drugged and kidnapped by a ring of evil people. Was she not spirited away in a car by strangers? Was she not placed in a bed with high sides, effectively imprisoning her? (A friend points out that considerable evidence supports her interpretation of events.) "By the way," Mom whispers to me on the phone, "the kidnappers are homosexuals. Maybe that's all right with you, dear, but it's certainly not *my* cup of tea." They were trying to involve her in their "shenanigans," in which patients and staff disappeared behind closed doors, from whence issued both laughter and moaning.

"You've got to get me out of here. They've got me in a prison bed."

"It's for your protection, Mom. They're trying to help you."

"No one will receive any help in here. They're trying to kill me. Maybe you're in on it too. If you won't get me out, I'll have to escape myself."

"Just hang on a bit longer. I'll come and take care of you." I live hours away, and with two jobs and a family, packing up to stay with her for a while will take a couple of days. But she does not wait. That night she tries to escape, a valiant act that involves squirming through the small gaps between the safety bars. She crashes to the floor hard, this time really breaking her hip.

Thus the hip-replacement surgery she bravely endures on an early Thursday morning, my brother and I and two grandchildren at her side. They'd taken her off the crazy-making meds prior to surgery, so she is once again sane. I'm now onto what's happening, so minutes after surgery, when the supervising doctor orders resumption of all three psychoactive meds, I find it out from a nurse who checks the chart for me. I argue with him, the youngest in a practice whose senior member is Mom's regular doctor, but the good Dr. Regan is not here and I'm dealing with this young guy full of good intentions and belief in the efficacy of pharmaceutical fixes, who clearly thinks it's OK to put a person on medication without informing family. I'm not against psychoactive drugs, but I'm wary. Finally I resort to the colloquial.

"Look, bottom line here, she wasn't nuts before, but she's nuts now."

"No, the medication doesn't *cause* paranoia, we're giving it to her to *treat* her paranoia." Clearly he believes he's dealing with an irrational daughter.

"Doctor, everyone knows that some antidepressants cause a few people to become suicidal. And when I took pills for an ear infection that made me dizzy, the side effect was more dizziness. She wasn't paranoid before, but now she is."

"Yes, and that's why we're giving her antiparanoia medication."

"No, it's the antiparanoia drug that's made her paranoid."

"No, she was paranoid before. It says so right *here*." He points to the psychiatric evaluation, which specifies mild paranoia, mild dementia symptoms, mild depression. So he's put her on the antidepressant, an antipsychotic, and one of the new memory-improvement drugs, also psychoactive. I don't know a lot about them, just enough to know that *they* don't know much about how the latter two work either—not the doctors, not even the researchers. Negative interactions are not uncommon. Friends with elderly parents who have been put on these new drugs are divided between those who swear by them and those who think they're toxic. I don't think this is the right time to experiment with my mother's mind. She's my mother, not his. But he's not listening, and I can't argue anymore, because Mom needs me to be there when she comes out of the recovery room.

I abandon my protests for one evening, during which someone adds Demerol to the stew of postoperative drugs that now total fourteen, the names of which a nurse lets me copy down, unauthorized, in Mom's hospital bathroom. By a day after surgery, she's raving nonstop about plots to brainwash her, it being clear that I have already been recruited, and now the lesbians have been joined by the Pentecostal Christians, strange bedfellows to be sure. All of this makes psychological sense to me—she's always been homophobic and probably unconsciously attracted to the idea, like many homophobes, and both of her dead husbands were ministers. Of course her mind is full of fear of lesbians, and of strict-interpretation Christian sects.

If all of this were not so disturbing, it would be funny. Now and then I manage a weak laugh, like when some guy in a polyester bowling jacket and ballcap walks by and she sinks down, telling me I must save her from him. "He's in on it too, you know," she says, shrinking under the covers. "Don't let him see me, he'll try to exert . . . mind control." She wags her gnarly index finger at me from under the covers as she says this, only her darting eyes and her finger peeking out.

But now the postsurgical Demerol starts to kick in, and she begins to hallucinate. I am alone with her in her room. I haven't had a lick of REM sleep in days. We've been here together on and off for two days, the cafeteria is closed, and the vending machine has maliciously stolen my last three bucks—who's paranoid?—so I'm hungry and there's no food. I am standing at the bottom of her bed when it begins.

"You have a fish flying through your hair, dear," she points out. "Can't you feel it? Who's that man in the corner?"

"What man?"

"The one in the raincoat." Her face darkens with suspicion. "You're not going to pretend you can't see him. Say there, missy—can you keep a secret?" She tilts her head and beckons me to her. There's a strange look in her eyes. Oh no. She is going to . . . to . . . confide in me.

"Sure," I answer. Uneasy. Curious, though. My mother does not talk like this.

"Well, it's about Louis." She refers to my stepdad, her second husband whom she divorced, who remained my dad until his death. When she married him, he brought his two kids, and she had her two. Together we formed a family that worked for us kids, though not for our parents, who went from being in love to being at each other's throats inside of two years.

"I wouldn't want him to know I'm telling you this," she cautions.

"I won't tell him, Mom." He's been dead for ten years.

"Well, I always felt like such a perfect ass that I failed at that marriage. I failed to make a good marriage and a family." In an instant, I understand what has never occurred to me before. For her generation, a failed marriage meant, in many respects, a failed life. I never knew she felt this way. In her normal state of mind with her defenses up (and they are always up), she'd never have said such things. "No, Mom, you didn't fail—you and Louis couldn't make it together. But your kids all did—we're still family—we're brothers and sisters; don't you know that?"

"Really?" she says. "Does it feel like that?"

"Yes, believe me, we all care very much for each other. Don't worry, Mom, you gave us a family and you gave us a dad. Louis was a wonderful father to us."

"I hope so, because I *have* felt like an ass all these years."

"But you mustn't. Please try to let that go now. It's sad that the marriage didn't work, you and Louis lost out, but we kids did fine."

"Well. OK." She is playing with the coverlet. She seems to be taking heart. I am trying not to cry, and I am not good at this—I normally go years, decades even, without weeping, but lately I am a sniveling mess.

"We're sisters, aren't we?" she whispers. "You're my very own sister, *and* you're my mother *and* you're my daughter."

"Yes, Mom, yes I am; I'm all those things." It's all true, nothing crazy about this part.

"But mostly, we're sisters now."

"Yes, we are." Now it's not the possibility of tears that unnerves me. I fear I am going to skip that phase altogether and simply wail.

"And we can tell each other anything. Is there anything you want to tell me?"

"No, Mom, I think you know it all."

"Is your, you know, relationship good with John?"

"Yes, Mom, it's just fine." OK, she's going for the smut now. I'll be OK.

"He doesn't have any . . . propensities I'd better be told about?" She's hopeful.

"Nope. The guy is pretty much without propensities." I am not stupid enough to tell my mother anything about sex, even under the influence of the most powerful drug of all, intimacy. And that's what this is, it's an end to the silence, it's intimacy between me and my mother, and it has not happened like this before. For the next hour or so, she sees colors, hears voices, laughs, comes up with odd memories. She tells me more secrets, ones I intend to keep.

But then a nurse is at the door with afternoon meds. As nice as this interlude has been, it's also been punctuated by flying animals, caves in the bathroom, the guy in the raincoat, and those kidnappers in their bowling jackets. Just before the nurse arrives, Mom has begun raving again about the lesbian/Christian kidnap ring. Maybe I owe this rare moment to the machinations of the medical community, but I don't want any more of it. Being fully psychotic and hallucinating can't be *good* for a barely postoperative old person, Timothy Leary be damned.

"No, no more pills now," I say, blocking the nurse's entry.

"But these are her medications. She has to have them."

"Not the ones making her crazy, she doesn't." I gesture at Mom, as if I were about to say, "Behold. See for yourself, a madwoman." And Nurse Nancy does behold. Nancy has the same name as my lifelong best friend, the one Mom hated when we were girls, because she thought we were up to no good together. (Also not paranoid. We *were* up to no good.) Immediately Mom says she will not put up with this, that I am in league with this woman, this Nancy, this nurse, this *ostensible* nurse; in fact, she does not think this is any nurse at all. She knows what we are up to and we won't get away with it.

"I see your true colors now," she says, pointing at me, her eyes narrowed slits in her extraordinarily young face—young because, as she has told me, she learned how not to smile or laugh, because it gives you wrinkles and lines. Thus her almost impassive lifelong facial expression. "You're not my sister at all, are you?"

"Oooh," says Nancy, who does remind me of my Nancy, "it's payback time. What did you do when you were a kid?"

"I hear you whispering," Mom says. "Don't think for one minute you're fooling *me*, girls, I'm onto your tricks." She nods and points from me to Nancy.

"Lots," I say to Nancy, "I did lots. I deserve this." Nancy says she cannot discontinue the meds without a doctor's orders. No medical man in sight. "Well, Nancy, you won't be giving her any meds at all then."

"But I have to, she really needs some of these. For clotting and inflammation."

"Not before I talk to a doctor about some of them," I say.

"Oh my Lord!" Mom cries. "What's happening to your face?" She gesticulates in my general direction. "You're a hundred years old!" I don't feel far from that. I feel like Ursula Andress in that film called *She,* just before she dissolves into a crone. "Honey, get a doctor, your face is falling off in chunks!" I feel my face. It's still there. I tell her so.

"No, no, no, you're bleeding from the holes in your face!"

"I'm not bleeding, Mom, believe me." I have not bled from any orifice in years. I have been prematurely postmenopausal for almost a decade.

"Hey! Hey, hey, HEY! Your forehead is coming off! Nurse, get her some help!"

"Yeah, Nancy, get me some help here. Can't you see my face is falling off?" She leaves, in search, I can only hope, of a doctor.

Now Mom is raised almost straight up, propped on an elbow. "You're a hundred years old, a hundred years old," she keens. "You're older than I am! And you're bleeding, dear, you're bleeding from the holes in your face. Can't you feel it?"

"No, I can't," I say, feeling my face, wondering if it might be true.

"Well, go in the bathroom and look in the mirror. For heaven's sake, child!"

I oblige, peering through the fluorescent lights that always make me dizzy. What I see is my sleepless countenance, weary and genuinely frightened for her now. "Not bleeding, Mom. My whole face is right here. And I'm OK. I'm only in my fifties. See?"

"No, your skin is coming off in your hand and you're a hundred years old and I hate to say it, dear," she adds in a cattily lucid aside, such as could occur only in a woman of her generation, "but you have *not* aged well. Not nearly as well as I have."

I laugh at this. She does not, for she was amused only momentarily before new horrors greeted her.

"Your right eye, it's blowing up like a golf ball! I always hated golf, never saw the use of it. Your uncles played golf. Your father played golf sometimes. Can't you feel that? It's coming right out of your head." I am standing in helpless fascination at the foot of her bed. She points, well to the side of my head. "It's there, your eye is *there* now."

"Exactly where do you see my eye?" Both of us are keenly interested in its migration.

"It's a full foot to the side of your head, attached by that cord. Doesn't that hurt? Oh!" She winces. "There goes another chunk of your face!" I'm now thinking of the corpse disintegration scene in *An American Werewolf in London*. There is little to do while waiting for a doctor to appear, but to try to understand exactly what she beholds.

"So is my eye, what, about *here*?" I point to the empty space next to my face. Too appalled now for speech, she gestures more to my right, her left. "Here?" I move my finger another six inches. She nods. "Ah," I say. "Well, what's *here* then?" I point to my real eye.

"It's empty, it's just a bloody socket." I have no idea what to do or say next, when suddenly my hero, Dr. Regan, her regular family doctor, appears at the door with his jaunty bow tie and his family-doctor bag of worn black leather that I always find comforting. He always looks like Marcus Welby.

"How are you, Janice?" he asks my mother, striding in and sitting on the edge of her bed. I think soon all will be well, for he will see she has taken leave of her senses. But in moments it becomes clear by the look on her face she has decided he's in on The Conspiracy, so with everything she's got, she pulls herself together. My mother has considerable powers of performance.

"Fine, just fine," she answers, "though I would like you to check this bandage."

"Sure, Janice, I'll do that as soon as I wash up here." He heads to the bathroom. Mom beckons me close and whispers, "Be careful, he's one of them now. Watch out."

"No, Mom, it's Dr. Regan. Tell him the truth. Tell him what you've been seeing."

"No, no," she hisses, "it would not be safe. They'll kidnap me again."

"So everything's fine, Janice?" Dr. Regan resumes his position on her bed.

"Oh, yes," she says. "I like your tie. You're looking quite spiffy today." Spiffy? The old girl is half flirting with the good doctor. Out of what hat did she pull this trick?

"Why, thank you," he says. "Now tell me more about how you're feeling," he continues, getting out his gear.

"I haven't had much pain at the surgical site, but it's very uncomfortable."

"Mom," I say pointedly, "I want you to tell Dr. Regan what you see when you—"

Dr. Regan holds a hushing hand toward me. "I'm asking your *mother* how she feels." This must be standard when adult children try to speak for their parents.

"My gown isn't on straight," she fusses, "but the meals are good." It goes on like this. "The surgeon was skillful, and I told him he has a rugged kind of good looks."

No plots? No lesbians? No mind control? I'm twitching by the time he says, "Well, then, let's give you your medications now." They're in a Dixie cuplet in his hand.

"No!" I squeak, lurching toward his hand as if it contained poison.

Dr. Regan admonishes me again. "*We* will talk after she takes her medications."

"No, just please wait a minute. Mom, I want you to look at me. I want you to tell Dr. Regan what you see when you look at me." I am hoping against hope that my eyes are not back in my head. "And I want you to tell him the truth. Because don't you think I need some help? And I can't get help if you don't tell the truth." Dr. Regan is poised over her, a half-full cup of water for the pills in his hand. He's clearly not going to wait much longer before dispensing them down her throat.

"Well," she begins, "I do wish you'd take a look at my daughter. She clearly needs some help." He looks at me. "As you can see," Mom continues, "her right eye is over there, and don't you think she has aged a great deal today? She's at least a hundred."

I smile broadly. I point to my eye. "Bloody socket here," I note.

He hesitates, taken aback. He glances from her to me, a puzzled frown forming on his face. Mom continues, "There's blood running down her face, and part of her face is missing."

Dr. Regan is staring at my face, processing her words, now registering a fair degree of cognizance that causes him momentarily to lose track of his wrist. He spills the little cup of water right down Mother's hospital gown.

She yelps and he dabs at her chest.

"I'll take care of this," I say sweetly, grabbing a towel. "Perhaps you might want to take a look at the three psychoactives and the Demerol on her chart? The ones I wasn't told she'd be put back on? The ones I keep asking for her to be taken off of? I have been trying to explain to your colleague for two days that she's having an allergic reaction."

Minutes later, he and I are in the hall speaking in low tones. Mom is inside the room behind the closed door, raving about the Christian/lesbian kidnappers, of which she is now doubly certain I am one of. He takes her off all psychoactives and strongly hints that he does not like their overuse. I am so relieved. When I ask how long they'll take to get out of her system, he says it should be a matter of a few hours, especially the ones that could, in interaction, cause this. He tells me he won't be here tomorrow, but not to worry, that everything will be all right.

When I get back to the hospital in the morning, Mom is sane, already her old unpleasant self, complaining of underlings who are not giving her proper service. "Did you see that aide who was just in here? I want you to report her to the authorities. She did not perform her duties adequately. I know my rights."

"Sure, Mom, right away." The day-nurse arrives with the meds tray while I am in the bathroom. When I emerge, she is giving Mom her cup of water and is about to empty the pills into Mom's hand. Glancing into the cup, I see a lot of pills.

"Excuse me," I say, "I need to see the list of pills you're about to give her."

She reads them aloud. All of the psychoactive medications are back on the list. "There's been some sort of mistake," I say. "Dr. Regan discontinued these."

"Yes," says the nurse, one I've never seen before, "but Dr. Regan is out of town today and his colleague reordered them this morning. And I see he upped the dosages." She used the younger doctor's name during this exchange, which I recognized immediately from my previous discussions with him, though I don't recall it now, and I have refrained from looking it up in my records.

"No, you can't give her these. I want to see the doctor."

"He's somewhere on his rounds, and I have to give these to her now."

"No, you don't, and trust me, don't try to talk me into this because it will not work. Just report that an uncooperative family member is refusing to allow you to do your job."

This brings the young doctor. We reenact our scene from two days ago. I very nearly put my hand on his shoulder, so sincere is he, so much does he believe in the accuracy of the psychiatrist's report. I've got enough friends in psychiatry to know how misplaced is his utter faith in this diagnostic language, based on one short intake interview. "I think you're making a mistake here," he opines and walks away, shaking his head. Such a nice man. Such good intentions. I am so angry I could smack him.

That night, alone in a hotel room, I begin to bleed, not from my face, but from the other end of my body, for the first time in many years. I gaze at the unaccustomed sight of fresh blood, entirely foreign, nothing like the blood of menstruation. *This is wrong blood,* I say aloud, to make myself know it. I might as well be bleeding from my eyes.

Two weeks later, I have minor gynecological surgery. I react badly to the anesthetic, and my pulse slows to twenty in recovery. Conscious, I watch as nurses and doctors react to a crisis. I know it involves me, and it is life-threatening, but I am calm, even when I hear directives to get more atropine into my intravenous tube. Now I understand how my mother could have managed to be so fundamentally calm, even when her mind showed her such apparitions. Once, I feel my face, to see if it is all there. It is. I feel unspeakably old.

But once I get home and crawl into bed, I feel like a kid who wants to be taken care of. I would like oatmeal with bananas. I would like ginger ale, like Mom used to bring me when I was sick. I'm still in bed, postoperative and pouting, when I begin reading the typescript of a novel my mother wrote over thirty years ago. I encounter this barely disguised autobiographical scene in which the heroine, Celeste, visits her mother Alanna in a hospital, after Alanna has had a stroke. Celeste is a stand-in for my mother, and Alanna for my grandmother.

> *There was her darling sick mother, pale and gaunt, sitting helplessly in a bed with high metal sides all around it. This first time, Alanna recognized her daughter. "Celeste, help me get out of here!" Celeste thought, "We start in the crib and sometimes we end up in it, too." The steel sides looked forbidding.*
>
> *"Mom, I can't—you were getting out of bed and hurting yourself. You must stay in bed now—I'm sorry."*
>
> *"Why, Celeste—help me!" Alanna protested pitifully.*
>
> *That was as lucid a moment as Celeste ever again saw in her mother.*

My mother is lucid again now, at least some of the time. She corrected my grammar the other day, and I could kiss her for it. I have not told her I was bleeding and needed a doctor. She already knows that.

Diana Hume George is the author of *The Lonely Other: A Woman Watching America*, and author or editor of a number of other books of poetry, essays, and literary criticism. She teaches in the Creative Nonfiction MFA program at Goucher College and codirects the Chautauqua Writers' Festival.

Foreign Bodies

Grace Talusan

Often, as an ophthalmologist, my father has to deliver bad news. He tells people what's wrong with their eyes and hands them some words to hold on to: astigmatism, cataracts, glaucoma, macular degeneration. After thirty years of practicing medicine, he expects his patients will receive the most difficult news with resistance and denial. The truth is painful: our bodies will let us down; our eyes will disappoint us.

I was there, photocopying insurance cards in his medical clinic, when he told an elderly woman she was legally blind. According to the National Association for the Visually Handicapped, the legally blind are defined as those "who test 20/200 or less in the better eye after the best correction, or have a field defect in which the widest diameter of the visual field is no greater than 20 degrees."

The blind woman was shocked. "But I can see fine," she insisted. She held her daughter's elbow, sobbing, as they trudged down the hallway to the waiting room. My father signed some official papers attesting to her blindness, as she was now entitled to certain government programs. The woman couldn't see any less than when she had walked into my father's office. In fact, the woman had probably been blind for quite a while before my father's words confirmed her suspicions.

Recently my father told me about the man who burst into tears when told that his child would need glasses.

"But all the kids at school will make fun of him," the man said. "Maybe we can wait until he's a little older and bigger."

With calm delivery and no judgment in his voice, my father answered, "Your child's vision is blurry. He can't see the board at school. He can't see a car coming when he crosses the street."

But the man who is the ophthalmologist, the one who always acts in his patients' best interest, is not entirely the same man who is my father.

Love obstructed my father's vision. Like the blind woman who didn't want to admit she was blind, in a moment when my father inhabited two identities at once, as an eye doctor and a grandfather, he denied the truth. His fear struck him mute.

August 18, 2005, finds me pressed against the picture window on the seventh floor at Massachusetts Eye and Ear Infirmary. The Charles River shimmers, and for a weekday morning there are a surprising number of sailboats gliding figure eights on its surface. It's a beautiful day, the kind of day that reminds us we must hold on to summer before it's gone, before the autumn forces us inside, to retreat to the warmth and to the loneliness of our televisions.

Ten adults crowd this hospital room, missing meetings and not returning phone calls and e-mails so that we can sit around this empty bed. We're waiting for my two-year-old niece, Joli, to return from emergency surgery to remove her right eye. An enucleation. The doctors are certain: it's cancer. Retinoblastoma. The malignant kind, the kind that can kill you.

My mother sits in a plastic chair, counting the hours in rosaries, fingering each bead with a Hail Mary or Our Father, around and around. In the spiritual equivalent of slipping cash to the hostess of an exclusive restaurant, my mother prays to her dead parents and siblings, begging them to whisper in God's ear and intercede on her behalf. Joli's other grandparents, the preacher and his wife, pray softly, and an occasional "praise God" or "in Jesus' name" rises to my ears. Joli's mother, my sister Liza, reads the latest *Harry Potter*, and Joli's father, Jorge, talks on the phone, telling and retelling the story for the hours we wait.

I notice Jorge's wearing the Superman T-shirt he wore on the day Joli was born, the one inked with Joli's newborn feet. It used to hang inside a box frame on the wall in his study, and I wonder about his decision to wear it. I see his loneliness and despair as he unhooks the frame from the wall, unpins the shirt from the frame, and pulls it over his head. These small actions are his attempt to create some luck.

As soon as he heard the news, my brother Jon took a flight from Maui, traveling across the Pacific then the continent. My other brother, Paul, a first-year medical student at Boston University, skips his classes to sit with us. Alonso, my boyfriend of a decade, waits here, too. My sister Mari, who is due to give birth any week now, calls us constantly from Los Angeles for updates.

But there's a noticeable and puzzling absence: my father, the ophthalmologist, and we act as if his absence proves the depth of his love for his granddaughter. My father must love Joli more than any of us, and that's why he's not here.

But I know the truth of why my father isn't here: he blames himself. If Joli dies because my father was silent, waiting too long before voicing his suspicions about the subtle, almost imperceptible changes to her eye that he, as an eye surgeon himself, was the only one of us in a position to interpret—if Joli dies because my father didn't say a word and the cancer finds the opportunity to burst from her eye and eat her brain and spinal cord—I will blame him too.

Reach back twelve hours, to the evening of August 17. On the seventeenth of every month since Joli's birth, my sister Liza has posed Joli with a stuffed Tigger and posted these photos to her baby blog. The baby blog meticulously documents firsts in Joli's life, which, considering she's just turned two, is almost everything. But on this day, the same day Joli was diagnosed with cancer, instead of merely marking her growth, the Tigger photo showed Joli's tumor. Joli's eyes were still dilated from her eye exam, and in the flash photography, the tumor in her right eye was obvious, unmistakable. Where normal red-eye reflex should have occurred, Joli's right eye revealed an opaque pearl.

In that night after first hearing of Joli's diagnosis of retinoblastoma (Rb), I learned of grandmother Pam Bergsma. Like many proud and enthusiastic grandparents, Bergsma took dozens of photographs of her grandson, Joey. Some photos were marred by red eye, which occurs when the red blood vessels in the retina reflect light, while others showed a cloudy white spot, similar in appearance to a cataract.

On her Web site, Bergsma said, "I was taking pictures of the tumor reflecting the light and did not know it. These pictures would have saved his vision and his life."

Since her grandson Joey died from retinoblastoma at age three in December 2000, Bergsma's mission has been to educate and alert people about what that mysterious white spot in a child's photo might signal, and to advocate for policy changes that include early screening for ocular diseases as part of routine well-baby exams. In the years since Joey's death, Bergsma has received many letters from people who say their child's life was saved because of one of her posters. Bergsma conducts regular seminars for health care professionals, and says nurses come by the hundreds, yet pediatricians, who have the tools and the authority to conduct the eye exams, rarely attend.

Despite her hard work, only in 2007 was Bergsma successful in filing The Infant Eye Care Bill in the state of Florida. "Joey's Bill" requires three eye exams as part of routine well-baby visits. In an e-mail, Bergsma tells me, "I have been begging for this simple exam for almost six years. This should not have happened to your niece. She should have her eye and her sight, and her precious life should never have been jeopardized." The routine enhanced eye exams Bergsma calls for add only ten seconds to the regular exam and cost pennies in eye dilation drops.

In fact, on the morning Joli was diagnosed, it took only seconds. The pediatric ophthalmologist just blinked into his ophthalmoscope before announcing to the shock of everyone, "Tumors. Looks like retinoblastoma." And just as quickly, my father, who was in the exam room chatting up his former colleague, spun around and left the room without saying a word. My father is the kind of man who can't let anyone know he cries. The team wanted to remove the eye immediately, but they weren't able to schedule surgery until first thing the next day.

My father didn't speak much for the rest of the day, nor did he leave the car to attend the flurry of appointments with specialists before my niece's operation the next morning. I was in the car alone with him when he said miserably, "We could lose her."

"Not lose her," I countered. "Just her eye. That's the worst-case scenario."

"Losing her eye," my father said, "is the least of our worries."

While in training for his ophthalmology specialty thirty years ago at Philippines General Hospital, my father had witnessed enough cases of Rb to fear it. Some of the parents he met had read the mysterious white glow from their toddler's eyes as a sign that their child was special, endowed with powers to divine the future or bring the family luck.

"Stupid," my father says. He watched their children die.

Once Joli was diagnosed, my sister Liza recalled moments in the past months where she saw a strange reflection from the night-light in Joli's right eye, like the glow of a cat's eye. But the conditions had to be just right, and Liza didn't see it all the time, so it didn't alarm her.

In 1869 only 5 percent of children diagnosed with retinoblastoma survived. The good news is that Joli was born in this century and in a developed country, where 97 percent of children survive Rb, though most with some visual impairment. If Joli had been born in the rural Philippines or anywhere medical care was out of reach, her survival rate would drop to 13 percent. At least one person if not dozens loved those children whether they were poor or not, and I think about all that pain, all those black holes ripped into the center of those families' lives.

Over a retinoblastoma listserv, I meet an adult survivor of Rb named Abby White, who founded the International Retinoblastoma Daisy Fund, an organization whose mission is to help children with Rb connect with care. Part of her work includes supporting research with an international team of advocates, scientists, and physicians. White helped develop the World Rb Registry and in an e-mail writes, "According to tumor registry data and calculations for those countries without reliable registries, based on birth rate, child mortality, and known prevalence rates for Rb, an estimated 9,000 children develop Rb each year. So while about 5,000 children are diagnosed with Rb per year, this figure doesn't include those children without access to health care who aren't counted. According to our estimates, roughly 4,000 children die of Rb without ever being correctly diagnosed or documented."

White was particularly moved when she heard about a girl from Botswana named Gorata Poonyane, Rati for short. Rati's parents were concerned about her eye when she was only four months old. White writes, "Although doctors suspected eye cancer at the time, delays in referral meant she was not seen by a pediatric ophthalmologist for another four months." Like Joli, Rati had her eye removed.

But Rati wasn't able to have chemotherapy, the treatment her physicians recommended, and after nineteen months, the cancer returned, bulging out from her eye socket. White learned of Rati's plight and arranged funding and treatment for her in Toronto. She received first-rate treatment, which included an autologous stem-cell treatment, and the cancer went into remission for a year, but while she was in treatment, suddenly it returned. Five months after her fourth birthday, after a trip to Disney World care of the Make a Wish Foundation, Rati died.

I want to ask her doctors in Africa, "How could you be so negligent with her care?" But I realize the question is larger than those few people who work within a system with limited resources. My question implicates all of us. Why such different outcomes when Joli's cancer was diagnosed in the final stage and Rati's cancer was discovered in the first few months of her life?

As the first grandchild in our family, Joli was the most photographed child in our family's history. That night after hearing Joli's diagnosis, my father studied hundreds of photos of her. "I didn't see it," my father said. "How could I not see it?"

Hindsight, right? In a handful of photos from the past four months, there were hints of the white spot in her eye, slight irregularities. Then over the summer, there it was while Joli blew out two birthday candles, while she sat with my father watching television after a summer cookout, while she posed indoors next to Clifford the Big Red Dog on an excursion to the Boston Children's Museum.

But Pam Bergsma is right. Clues are not enough. An eye exam in a darkened room with an ophthalmoscope as part of Joli's routine checkups would have caught the gooey tumors as they started to gather and grow. Instead, for months, the cancer cells on her retina grew, until there were so many cancer cells they detached her retina, blinding her in that eye, and none of us knew. And we'd been taking photos of the cancer for months. One eye gone.

The doctors explain: humans adapt. Children are especially good at adapting.

We didn't know how much we needed Joli until she came into our lives. When Joli was a year old, my sister Liza and my brother-in-law Jorge moved in with my parents in order to save money for a house. My parents were delighted. For almost a decade after their five children had left the nest, their house had been empty. Even Sashi, our family dog of seventeen years, had died and given my parents one less thing to argue about. There were rooms full of our old clothes that my parents didn't even go into anymore. The first time I visited my parents' house after Joli moved in, I was walking up the green-carpeted stairs and found one fuzzy pink sock, then a plush rattle. I heard laughter. Effusive. Explosive. Joyous. It had been so long.

Joli performs daily miracles we can't live without: she's thrown open the metal bulkhead door in the cellar where my father hoards his love. She shines herself at us and says, "I love you."

During that first year at my parents' house, one day a week Joli was mine. I don't have children of my own and thought it would be fun to pretend. I would leave my apartment before 7 a.m. so I could be the first person to greet Joli when she awoke. So it was I who performed the morning rituals of diaper change and warm milk bottle and snuggling. My name was one of her first words, and her parents taught her the Filipino word for aunt, *tita*. As her vocabulary grew, I was *Tee* Grace, then *Tee Tah* Grace; and then she sang my name into a birdcall like the northern bobwhite, *Tee Ta Grace.*

We attended a Mommy and Me–type music class together, and I pretended to be her Mommy. The first time I brought her there she was so anxious she vomited. The next couple of classes she sat on my lap and held my arms around her like a scarf as she watched the other children dance and sing. Then one day she jumped out of my lap as soon as Jane began to play the guitar, and before I knew it, Joli was leading the toddler mosh pit.

My day a week that year with Joli provided some of the best times of my life. We threw an entire box of cereal onto the living room floor by the handful and let her dog Gordie, the 170-pound Presa Canario, clean it up. We simulated snow by emptying a container of baby powder in her bedroom. We tossed pizza dough into the air and cracked eggs against the counter and spooned soil with ice cream scoops into seedling trays on the coffee table. After our day together, I'd feed her, then bathe her. I'd rock her on my belly and tell her a story, then continue retelling it, until Joli stopped saying, *Again, again, again.*

As the daughter of an ophthalmologist, I was constantly aware of my eyes. The world I knew was riddled with dangers to the eye. My father prohibited us from throwing snowballs or eating lollipops or filling out crossword puzzles in the car or letting the dog lick our face. *One of his teeth might pierce your eye.*

I learned to respect the raw power of drinking straws, pencils, metal clothes hangers, baseballs, pencils, and tree branches. When I started working for my father at age eight, earning a few pennies for each medical chart I completed by pasting in multicolored chart numbers, he told me about foreign bodies. "Foreign bodies—dust, metal shavings, wood chips," he explained, "prevent people from seeing. Sometimes they make your eye infected. Sometimes they can make you blind." But at eight, I imagined miniature men in ethnic costumes kicking as my father plucked them from the whites of his patients' eyes.

My father saved up stories from the hospital and transformed them into directives: *Never let a parrot sit on your shoulder. I don't care how well you think you know him.* One of his patients liked to feed her parrot almonds that she balanced on her lips. One time the parrot mistook her eye for an almond.

Don't carry pencils, sharpened end up, in your shirt pocket. Watch out for corners on bookshelves and tabletops; better yet, only buy furniture with rounded edges. Avoid long stem roses, popsicles, high heel shoes, and the hardcover editions of books. No jumping on the bed—look what happened to your brother.

My brother Jon was almost two when he fell from the bed, hitting his eye on the corner of the wooden headboard. It's taken decades for me to learn the details: how my father carried Jon through the emergency room of the hospital where he worked, past the waiting room and nurses' station. He sat my screaming brother on a bed and pulled the yellow curtain around them. My father didn't trust the resident on call; he apparently didn't trust anyone but himself to hold the sharp points of the syringe, the threaded needle, and surgical scissors close to Jon's eye. My mother helped hold my brother down. My father sobbed as he sewed the stitches, but his hand was steady and careful. He understood how important the face is to human interactions, how a scarred and disfigured eye could impact his son's future. The pink scar drawn underneath Jon's left eyebrow is a faded testament to a close call and my father's expert hands.

But now, with Joli's diagnosis, I feel robbed. I want to tell my father, "You taught me to be afraid of pens and lollipops and snowballs and rosebushes and everything else in the world when all this time the danger was inside of us, close to home."

When we tell the story of Joli's cancer to new people, my father, the ophthalmologist, is the hero. It was he who first noticed that Joli's right eye was slightly misaligned. During Easter holidays, I heard murmurs about strabismus or lazy eye, and a month later my father began to share his suspicions regularly to any of us who would listen. At a Mother's Day meal, my cousin Rod, who is also a physician, admitted that he thought Joli was going cross-eyed.

Despite all the talk, no one was alarmed. We didn't want to consider that she might be imperfect; we didn't think her misaligned eyes could threaten anything but her looks. Silent alarms were firing in my father's head—*Misaligned eyes! These could be symptoms of a rare eye cancer*—but he wasn't able to voice his fears. The malignant cells went on dividing.

My oldest sister was married that Memorial Day weekend, and all through the festivities, I noticed my father placing one hand, then the other in front of Joli's eyes. He would sneak his hand around from behind and try to cover Joli's eye, but she was a toddler. She would swat it away.

"Leave her alone," I said. "She doesn't like that."

Months later, after Joli's cancer was diagnosed, my father, in a story he can't stop telling, a story that implicates him again and again—*Why didn't I know?*—tells me that he was doing that annoying hand trick to check Joli's visual field. "But she saw my hand," my father said. "She saw it."

I understand what he needs—forgiveness, relief from culpability. "You couldn't have known," I said. And it's true. Without a proper exam with the right instruments, he couldn't have. But I wish he had been able to speak up about his concerns. I wish he had said, "I doubt it's anything serious, but I've noticed Joli's right eye is wandering to the side. It's my professional recommendation that you take her to a doctor."

But he wouldn't ever have said that. My father, the ophthalmologist, sends his patients to other eye experts when he understands his limitations as a general eye doctor. "I have to send you to Boston," my father says to his patients. "They can take care of you there."

The irony is that my father, although he is doctor, doesn't believe in going to the doctor. His medicine cabinet is full of prescriptions he's written for himself—antibiotics for sore throats and topical creams for his eczema. (At least, I think it's eczema; he's never been to a dermatologist to know for sure.) He has health insurance, and plenty of his physician friends would see him for free—that's not the problem.

The problem is he understands far too well how disease waits for every body, and part of him still believes that not acknowledging there's something wrong will make it go away.

My father's not unusual among his friends—cardiologists who smoke and drink, psychiatrists and gynecologists who fall asleep in the middle of a weekend mah-jongg and drinking binge. They believe their status and training as doctors make them exempt from the body's limits. One colleague, who had two children under the age of six, was covered in bruises and so fatigued she was crawling up the stairs. The doctors confirmed what she already knew, leukemia, and she was dead in three months.

By the time another friend, a psychiatrist, was diagnosed with lung cancer the only option left was palliative care, a pain-free dream he slipped into for several weeks, and then he was gone. Probably the outcomes would have been the same for these two of his friends; maybe early diagnosis wouldn't have bought them more time. But that isn't what upsets me. My doctor father neglects his body. He's taught me to feel this way about my body, and I have habits of punishing it I've had to work very hard to undo: smoking, over- and undereating, over- and underexercising, sitting so still my legs fall asleep, holding my urine until I'm in pain.

Come June 2005, all five of my brothers and sisters, their significant others, my parents, and anyone else in my niece's life weighed in with their opinions: does she or doesn't she have a lazy eye?

"Call it amblyopia," I said. "'Lazy' is so judgmental."

None of us wanted to consider that my niece wasn't perfect, that there may have been something about her appearance that could turn people off. Many times, we've poked fun at those with misaligned eyes: the popcorn vendor at the cinema, the clerks at the town library, the odd colleague with poor social skills. We laughed, "Which eye do we look at when we're talking to him?" Children are cruel; adults, even crueler.

In early July a friend revealed that she had surgery as a toddler to correct her wandering eye. Now her eyes are perfectly aligned, and this information gave me courage to insist. I told my sister, "Get some medical advice about Joli's eye from an ophthalmologist who isn't also her grandfather."

I started researching cross-eyes and lazy eyes. I found out that waiting too long before seeking treatment can result in the eye's becoming permanently blind. There are all kinds of solutions—surgery to repair the muscles that cause the misalignment or exercises or eye patching. But it was clear to me that waiting could produce irreversible vision loss.

I was overstepping a line. Never interfere between parent and child. It's none of my business; her parents know what's best for her. I'm just the aunt; I don't have any children of my own and probably never will. Keep my mouth shut.

But for Joli, I found courage. I couldn't afford to love blindly. So I insisted. I pushed. I broke past the silence and spoke up on my niece's behalf.

Almost five months had passed from when the question began to form in my father's mind. The tumors grew very quickly, and in that time Joli's eye went blind. There's no guarantee doctors could've saved that eye even if they had found the cancer early, and in a way, finding the cancer at its final stage was a blessing. Now there was no choice but to remove the eye. Maybe if it had been caught earlier, they would have been tempted to save the eye through radiation or other treatments that can be painful and disfiguring. But timing is everything—if the Rb cells had been allowed to escape and tumors were found outside of the eye, Joli's survival rate would've dropped below 10 percent.

August 18, 2005, before Joli's surgery, after Liza and Jorge dress Joli in the surgical gown, someone takes a last family photo with Joli's right eye intact. Joli is wearing a yellow gown that opens in the back and thick hospital socks with rough treads on the feet. Her thick curls aren't brushed, and she's crying.

When Joli's parents leave her on the operating table, they still must ask, "This isn't a mistake? You sure it's my kid who has cancer?"

After surgery, scans and biopsies and spinal taps are performed; bone marrow is mined. For ease of access to Joli's vascular system, a plastic port, like a piece of uncooked ziti, is hidden under the skin next to her left nipple. Her baby-smooth skin is bruised from the needles, raw from bandage adhesive that stays stuck for days.

After surgery, Joli doesn't speak or even cry. Liza lays in bed and Joli settles underneath her mother's breasts as if she's an enraged squatter trying to move back inside the only home where she ever felt safe. If anyone tries to kiss or touch Joli or if Liza readjusts her position, Joli shrieks like a wild animal. She has white bandages over her right eye, protruding like a fist.

Immediately after surgery, we discover that no sign of cancer has been found in the other eye, and that on first glance, there are no obvious signs of spreading—all good news.

As we wait for Joli's anesthesia to wear off, we sit together in this hospital room and wait, looking out the window so we don't have to look at each other. We eat soup and drink coffee. We make excuses about why my father, the ophthalmologist, isn't here for his granddaughter's eye surgery. We understand that like all of us, he's doing the best he can.

We cover our mouths with our hands and whisper the story into our cell phones, retelling the narrative again and again to anyone who'll listen, ending the variation on a theme by saying in one way or another the words we hope are true: "Everything will turn out fine. We'll get through this."

Grace Talusan was following in the footsteps of her physician parents until her last premedical school requirement: Organic Chemistry II. Despite her best efforts, she failed and finally admitted that she really wanted to be a writer. She earned an MFA in Fiction from the University of California, Irvine, and currently teaches at Grub Street Writers in Boston.

You Have the Right to Remain Silent

Pamela Skjolsvik

The message was eerily familiar, dreadfully self-important, and delivered in a monotone. "This is a call from a federal penitentiary. To accept this call . . ." I know, I know. I hesitantly pressed the 5 button, perturbed that I would have to listen to yet another call that revolved around my soul's perilous state, or the hell that awaited me for not accepting Jesus Christ as my personal savior.

"Pizza Hut!" I answered, as chipper and bright as I could muster. My brother was silent, but I could hear his labored breathing, as the monotone voice continued its grave warning.

"Hello? Is anybody home? Time's a-tickin'."

Silence.

"Pamela, I just got the results back from my biopsy. It's not good."

I walked to the porch, lit a cigarette, and stalled for time.

"I'm dying." His voice cracked.

"What do you mean you're dying?"

"I've got stage 4 cirrhosis."

"Oh, Jesus."

Brad sighed exhaustedly at my uncanny ability to use the Lord's name in vain whenever we spoke.

"What are they going to do? Do you get to go to a hospital or something?"

"No. The doctor said it is too advanced for treatment. I've spent most of my life behind bars, I've got one more year to go, and the sad thing is, I'm probably going to die in here."

Since I was five years old, Brad was either in juvie or serving time in the big house. Recidivism could have been his middle name. He was the quintessential black sheep of the Johnson clan, while the other three kids in our family were either gray or severely mottled. As a teen, Brad was always in trouble with the law—robbery, car theft, burglary—and it was not unusual to see police cars parked in front of our house with their lights flashing. If there was a crime in Fargo, Brad was suspect numero uno. My father attributed Brad's criminal behavior to the ingestion of lead-based paint chips as a baby. Now, how could a mostly absent father who made a living gambling and a mother teetering on the verge of a nervous breakdown have had anything to do with his criminal behavior?

I barely knew my older brother the first time I ventured to see him in Folsom Prison, where he was stuck, for shooting not a man in Reno just to watch him die but a cop in Ventura during a high-speed car chase. I was twenty-one and living in San Francisco when I realized that he was only three hours away by car. I didn't go to visit him out of some great desire to reconnect, but more out of curiosity and to prove to my family that my fleece was still as white as snow. After a background check, I was cleared to go. I made sure not to wear jeans, "gang colors" or a T-shirt with any words on it. I woke up early and drove a rented car to the lovely town of Represa, situated in the heart of the sweltering Sacramento Valley.

The waiting area was packed, mostly with overweight, dentally challenged women and their small children who scampered about the room, high on sugary snack food from the vending machine. I felt alone and uncomfortable in that waiting room, like I was somehow on trial with these women whose bad choice of husband or boyfriend brought them here. He's just my brother, I wanted to inform them, in a casual, offhand way. I didn't choose him. Can't you tell by my smart outfit and my carefully styled hair that I'm nothing like him? But the guards' treatment of all visitors upon check-in made it clear we were guilty by association, familial or otherwise, and it was no use to argue the point. A young, intimidating female guard called my group, and we boarded the bus to New Folsom. With just a roll of quarters and my ID, I felt naked.

After passing through a metal detector, we were brought into a large gray room with a happy meadow mural on one wall where you could have your souvenir picture taken. *"I went to Folsom Prison and all I got was this lousy photo,"* I imagined telling my friends. The room was filled with industrial tables and chairs that all faced the front of the room, where a desk and several guards sat eyeing us like a bunch of errant cattle.

I sat down at the front table. *"Look at me! I have nothing to hide, here I am right in the front row!"* I wanted to flash the armed guards a knowing look to indicate that I was indeed on their side, and there was no need to worry. After five minutes, the inmates streamed in, dressed in dark crisp blue jeans and pressed work shirts. Brad saw me immediately and sauntered over to the table looking like a vision of health, with tanned skin and a muscular physique. The last time we had seen each other was during Christmas after his first release from the "pen." Back then, I was a frizzy-haired, insecure thirteen-year-old, and here I was now, an insecure full-grown woman with better hairstyling products. We reminisced about the past, ate candy, and sipped soda, while guards circled the room warning overly smoochy couples to cool off. Soon, the four hours were up and I drove back home feeling like a super-dee-duper nice gal.

Those visits at Folsom continued for five years, until Brad was transferred to the U.S. Penitentiary in Florence, Colorado, to serve his federal sentence, a welcome respite from the dreary thirteen years he had spent in Folsom. The food was better, there was more freedom, and the living conditions were like the Ritz-Carlton compared to his former digs. But, within a year of his transfer, he began to experience a sharp, gnawing pain in the area of his liver. He made an appointment with the prison doctor after a friend on the outside encouraged him to get a liver panel run. The test was performed, but there was no follow-up with the doctor concerning his test results. After the pain subsided, he eventually chalked the whole episode up to gas or stress or just getting older.

Three years went by and he didn't give that test a second thought until his cellmate was diagnosed with hepatitis C. Brad could hardly believe that his cellie, "who looked so healthy," had a deadly disease. Because HIV and hep-C testing were available to all inmates, Brad went in for a blood draw. When the doctor confirmed the positive result, Brad was shocked to learn he had a life-threatening disease and didn't even know it. The doctor flipped through Brad's medical records and casually stated, "Oh yeah. You tested high for enzymes back in '97." Nothing was done. No treatment. No information. To quell Brad's anxiety and answer his questions, a fellow inmate lent him a dog-eared copy of *Hepatitis C: The Silent Killer.*

At that point, my relationship with my brother had become strained. Brad had found God and I was his reluctant congregation of one. Before his conversion, Brad and I had been on friendly, brother-sister terms. I wrote him weekly and often sent him books and care packages to help kill the time in his six-by-nine-foot cell. But after he found God, Brad became judgmental of me. I was no longer a Good Samaritan on my way to earning a good-deeds patch. From his Christian fundamentalist point of view, I was the lowest of the low—spiritual, yet a nonbeliever of religious dogma. From an intellectual perspective, I understood Brad's need for religion as a way to cope and to find forgiveness for his sins, but I found it odd that the man who had turned him on to religion had been convicted of cutting up his girlfriend, stuffing her remains into a Samsonite bag, and throwing her into the river.

Since Brad's world now revolved around serious religious study and the even more serious state of his health, and I couldn't—or, should I say, wouldn't—agree with the religious beliefs he spouted forth in every phone call to me, I hooked him up with the National HCV Prison Coalition, which provided him with a newsletter about hepatitis C.

Brad was not alone: According to the coalition's Web site, www.hcvinprison. org, "It is estimated that between 25 percent to 40 percent of inmates incarcerated in state prison settings are infected with hepatitis C." Shared needles and the exchange of bodily fluids between inmates mean that someone could enter prison and unknowingly receive a death sentence if he didn't "keep his nose clean." Furthermore, according to the Centers for Disease Control, "the rapid turnover of the incarcerated population, especially in jails, and the suboptimal funding of correctional health and prevention services, often limits the correctional system in providing both curative and preventive care." Because of the lack of funding, meeting the criteria for treatment is akin to winning the lottery. Guidelines, even those adhered to by the prison system, are just that, guidelines, and that's if you know you have the disease. Many don't, as the disease is often asymptomatic, and screening for the disease is offered on a routine intake basis in only a handful of prisons.

Reading up on the disease made it abundantly clear to Brad that he needed to have a liver biopsy done to assess the damage. Doing that on the outside is one thing, but within the prison system, it is a bureaucratic nightmare. He was told that in order to qualify for a biopsy, he would need to have three panels done three months apart and that his liver enzymes would have to be triple the normal level in order to qualify. Brad waited it out, and with each successive test, his enzymes continued to rise. Since he now had a basic understanding of the disease and its effects on his liver, each day without treatment was interminable. At the end of this tormented trial, instead of getting a biopsy, he was transferred to another high-security federal prison in Greenville, Illinois.

During this time, our weekly correspondence on yellow legal pads stopped, the books I sent were given to other inmates, and the rare phone calls I did receive from Brad were filled with more religious preaching than a Sunday sermon. After hearing how disillusioned and evil I was, and not liking it very much, I checked my caller ID whenever the phone rang. But after the sad and desperate phone call in 2002, with the news that the prison had finally allowed a biopsy and then denied him treatment, I knew Brad needed me, or at least my Internet connection. The devil on my shoulder wanted me to tell him to give his old pal Jesus a call, but being the do-gooder sister that I am, I decided to help.

I wrote numerous letters to senators and congressmen in Illinois, the Bureau of Prisons, lawyers willing to take on a pro bono case, the warden, and Dr. Ben Cecil, a doctor who specialized in the treatment of hepatitis C and was known for his activism regarding inmate medical care. When no one returned my calls, I sent flowers, faxes, and e-mails, to gain their attention. In return, I received form letters, vacuous e-mails, and shrugged shoulders. I researched all aspects of the disease and the various treatment options and mailed them to Brad in thick manila envelopes. For his part, Brad filed a BP9, an administrative remedy form, to demand treatment. The prison's physician told him they didn't treat cirrhotic patients on the inside or the outside, that it was useless and that the drug used in the treatment, interferon, would probably kill him.

Brad called me several times a week to check my progress. Once again, it was becoming increasingly difficult to answer the phone. His life was in my hands, and I rarely had any news to offer that would ease his torment. If I hadn't realized it in the beginning, it was becoming glaringly clear that the people who could actually do something to help him were unwilling to do so. I can only surmise from their lack of action that in their minds he wasn't worth saving. He was a faceless number, a habitual criminal who'd shot at, though not killed, an officer of the law. He'd escaped from jail twice and he'd probably contracted the virus from illicit drug use while incarcerated. I began to think of my own prejudices. Would I want my tax dollars spent on treating a child molester, a murderer, a rapist? Probably not. But he was my brother, the one we weren't supposed to talk about, for fear of having his actions taint our own reputations as responsible law-abiding citizens. But regardless of how I felt about him, or how he felt about me, he was a human being who was suffering and deserved medical attention.

Just when I was about to give up hope, the National Institutes of Health (NIH) released a new standard of care for the treatment of hepatitis C patients. In Brad's case, it couldn't have come at a more fortuitous time. He was now considered a candidate for treatment, at least by general health care standards. I printed the full report and sent it to Brad with the hope that this information would help him get treated.

Since the NIH, to which the Bureau of Prisons adhered regarding inmate care, supported his case for treatment, and Brad was too outspoken and informed with stacks of statistics to be casually ignored, the prison doctor decided to treat him. As a requirement for treatment, Brad went to see a psychologist to determine his mental state, as interferon can cause severe depression. After receiving a clean bill of mental health, he began the combination therapy of ribavirin and pegilated interferon. Every Friday night, Brad marched down to the infirmary and stood in the pill line to receive a loaded hypodermic needle, which he injected himself. Throughout the yearlong course of treatment, Brad experienced insomnia, able to sleep some nights for only an hour, constant nausea, and general weakness, but no depression. Midway through the treatment, the doctor doubled the dose of interferon, and Brad's viral load plummeted to zero. At completion of the treatment, in December 2003, the virus had been eliminated from his body. One month later, Brad was released from prison after serving twenty years.

When we pulled into the Howard Johnson's lot in Colorado Springs, rain was pouring like mad. Spotting Brad's newly acquired gray Volvo, I unrolled my window and yelled, "Follow us." I figured my husband Erik and I would treat my culinary-deprived brother to a steak dinner at the ever-popular, family-friendly Outback Steakhouse. We dashed from our cars into the packed restaurant. It was Friday night, and we had an hour-long wait. This was going to be weird.

Brad looked pale, skinny, and drawn; his once very athletic 6' 4" body had curled into itself. His hair was thinning, and I could tell he was nervous. Since it's always easier to pay attention to children than to full-grown adults with chips the size of New Jersey on their shoulders, Brad paid attention to my two kids, like a doting uncle. When he finally turned to me, I half expected him to drop to the floor in that crowded waiting area and kiss my feet for all I'd done. When he smiled at me without a word, I decided to get the inevitable conversation flowing.

"So, Mom says you found a church here. What kind is it?" I asked in a light-hearted, fun tone.

"It's Presbyterian. Not that you'd know anything about it. Not all Presbyterians are the same," he replied.

"But don't they all serve the same purpose?" I questioned.

He quickly turned his attention back to my kids. I didn't press the point, as I had no desire to get into a discussion about religion. I knew little about the Bible, and Brad's careful examination of its contents for the last eight years would only result in a debate I was ill equipped to engage in.

When I removed my daughter Lola's jacket, revealing a pink Paul Frank skull-and-crossbones T-shirt, Brad couldn't keep his eyes off it. I hadn't thought when I dressed her that morning, but now I realized I had made a horrible mistake, and I just might burst into flames at any moment. Brad shifted uncomfortably on the bench while we waited. I realized in that half hour of uncomfortable silence that I was an appalling person in his eyes—no religion, and death emblazoned on my daughter's shirt. My efforts to help save his life were apparently trivial in comparison to my children's fashion choices.

I was relieved when we were seated and the food arrived. There was only so much "Let's avoid the pink elephant T-shirt" small talk I could take. Brad held his fork like a shovel and scooped up his salad, steak, and potato as if he was competing in a speed-eating race. When he finished before all of us, he scrutinized Lola eating her steak.

"You like steak?" he asked her in a voice people without children use to speak to them; high-pitched, singsongy, and syrupy.

"Yep," she said, dipping a small piece of meat into a puddle of A-1 sauce.

"Do you eat it a lot?" he pressed.

"Yep," she replied, blissfully unaware of the implications of such a statement.

"Actually, she likes macaroni and cheese the best," I added. I didn't want "materialistic child spoiler" added to my list of unspeakable sins.

We ended the night playing Monopoly at the house where Brad was staying. Brad was the dog, Erik was the top hat, and I was the car and the banker. With the game as our focus, Brad's old competitive spirit revived, and it clearly pained him that I was the high-rolling kingpin of the game. But then I landed on Chance. I picked up the orange card with dramatic flourish, as Brad anxiously waited to see the outcome. With karmic justice of the board game variety, I was instructed to "Go directly to jail. Do not pass Go. Do not collect $200." Brad looked at me and smiled.

"Don't worry, I'll come visit," he said and casually rolled the dice.

The fact that my brother was treated for hepatitis C while he was incarcerated was quite unusual. According to Dr. Ben Cecil, "One third of prisoners are infected with HCV, and less than 1 percent are treated because of the expense." That Brad remains free of the hepatitis C virus is even more amazing. His recovery is exceptional, as his genotype, 1A, is considered one of the most difficult to treat. He happily resides in Colorado Springs, where he is a successful carpenter, just like Jesus. Like 15 percent of American citizens, he is uninsured and probably never will be. His faith has never wavered, and he remains a devoted and active member of his church.

Our relationship, like that of most brothers and sisters, has its ups and downs, but lately we're more likely to argue about cell phone providers than spiritual salvation. I'd like to think that my involvement led to my brother's treatment and recovery, and perhaps it did. The Lord works in mysterious ways.

Pamela Skjolsvik lives in southwest Colorado with her husband and their two children. "You Have the Right to Remain Silent" is her first published piece.

See the Difference

Sue William Silverman

Clostridium difficile (klo-STRID-ee-um dif-uh-SEEL) is a bacterium that causes diarrhea and more serious intestinal conditions such as colitis.
—Centers for Disease Control (CDC)

After the death of my therapist in May 2005, followed by that of my cat in August, I wait. Not that I'm overly superstitious—but *don't* bad things happen in threes? So when amorphous, ghostly pains whisper through my lower abdomen, I fear I'm entering my own deadly portal. On October 19 I schedule an appointment with my doctor, her practice only ten minutes from my house in Grand Haven, Michigan. Dr. Sharon Fields pokes my stomach. She shakes her head: no grapefruit-sized tumor. She performs a Pap smear since I'm due for one anyway. "*Here's* the problem," she says, diagnosing a vaginal infection on the spot, without awaiting lab results. She prescribes an antibiotic, clindamycin, 300 mg capsules to be taken twice daily for a week. After leaving her office, vaguely satisfied I'll survive this relatively mild diagnosis—that *I* won't be the third in a fateful series—I stop at the pharmacy to fill the prescription at 10:30 in the morning.

At home I swallow the first turquoise pill, the color of a chlorinated, antiseptic pool of water. I'm convinced a pill wearing such a delectable, albeit chemically colored, jacket will cure me. I don't read the warning label. I rarely do, since pharmaceutical companies tend to list every conceivable side effect from hangnail to death. How can you tell? I simply trust my physician. I don't notice, therefore, that clindamycin "should be used only for serious infections because infrequently there are severe, rarely fatal, intestinal problems (pseudo-membranous colitis) that can occur."

And then I get sick.

On Saturday, October 29, ten days after starting the antibiotic regimen, I awake to a warm western Michigan morning. I also awake to mild intestinal distress. But since the evening before, my partner Marc and I celebrated his birthday by dining out, perhaps I have a touch of food poisoning. Or maybe a spice disagreed with me. Since I don't feel too poorly, Marc and I go for a walk, enjoying one of the final days of sunshine before the veil of a Midwestern winter descends. We stroll the quiet streets of Grand Haven before heading to the library. But here, amid the stacks, I weaken. I rest on a chair while Marc carries our books to the checkout desk. Walking home, the muscles in my legs seem to soften. They feel unmanageable, wayward, drunk. My black clogs, which usually clomp on pavement, now listlessly drag. I'm too tired to lift my feet. Exhaustion flares behind my eyes. I want to be in bed. Asleep.

Community Hospital, October 30

Clostridium difficile are diseases that result from *C. difficile* infections such as Colitis, more serious intestinal conditions, sepsis, and rarely death.

—CDC

"What're your symptoms?" Dr. Larson asks, after I'm admitted to the emergency room.

I consider mentioning Randy, my therapist, who died of heart failure in his early fifties, and Quizzle, my cat, dead at eighteen of lung cancer. I consider mentioning fate—that I'm ill simply because bad luck occurs in groups of three, whether the catastrophes are plane crashes or mysterious illnesses.

In fact, I wasn't the least surprised to find myself bundled into the car at six o'clock this morning, Marc driving us the five blocks to the emergency room along deserted Sunday streets. Last evening, collapsed in bed, wearing a sweatshirt and kneesocks to protect my diminishing body—making trip after trip to the bathroom, nineteen strides from bed to toilet, one way—I was afraid to sleep, convinced I'd die if I let down my guard. At any rate I *couldn't* sleep, egesting what seemed at least a month's worth of food. At times I drifted in an opaque haze, gazing at—if not actively watching—the Turner Classic Movie cable channel all night, beginning with *South Pacific*. After that, I time-traveled through a midnight film noir stupor, movies reeling one into the next, indistinguishable.

Between movies, I self-diagnosed various ailments with which I might be afflicted. The litany began when I (belatedly) read the warning label on the phial of clindamycin: "pseudomembranous colitis." The list expanded when I Googled "diarrhea" on my laptop, an instant link to a World Wide Web of disorders.

"I took this antibiotic," I now say to Dr. Larson. I hand him the clindamycin warning label.

He nods. "I've seen this before." He explains that a pseudomembranous colitis infection is caused by *C-diff.* bacteria, short for *Clostridium difficile*. "It's nasty stuff," he adds. "We'll run some tests, start an IV. You're probably dehydrated."

I lie on the hospital bed in the emergency room, watching transparent yellow fluid drip into my vein. Still early, it's relatively quiet. Small bleeps in the distance, perhaps a machine breathing life into a body. . . . Randy suffered a heart attack in his office, but I don't know if he died immediately or whether an ambulance rushed him to the hospital. With Quizzle, I asked the vet to come to my house to put her to sleep. She was already thin with cancer; I thought she'd be more comfortable fading away on her kitty condo beside her favorite window. Now, I want to doze, but the emergency room's searchlight-voltage fluorescent lights preclude rest. Also, I must roll the IV pole back and forth across the corridor to the bathroom. My body has a will of its own. It desires to be lighter, more deficient.

"The test is negative for *C-diff.*," Dr. Larson says about an hour later. "But that doesn't mean a whole lot. This is one of those tests that frequently shows a false negative."

He prescribes fourteen antibiotic metronidazole pills, 500 mg each, plus dicyclomine for cramping. "Stay on the BRAT diet—bananas, rice, applesauce, toast—for a week. Come back if you have additional symptoms."

Community Hospital, November 2

C. difficile symptoms include:
    Watery diarrhea (at least three bowel movements per day for two
        or more days)
    Fever
    Loss of appetite
    Nausea
    Abdominal pain/tenderness.

—CDC

"What're your symptoms?" Dr. Harkness, another ER doctor, peers at me.

For the past three days, I have nibbled only bananas, rice, applesauce, and toast. Small sips of Gatorade. But my body feels threatened even by bland food, impolitely rejecting it. I explain what I've been through the last three days. "I'm exhausted," I add.

"We'll hook up an IV and run more lab tests," he says, glancing at my chart.

"What if it's *not* a *C-diff.* infection?" I ask.

"That'll be good."

"But what're the other options?" I ask.

"Maybe Crohn's disease," he says.

"But isn't that bad? Worse?" But he disappears before the question is fully asked, much less answered. From the little I know, Crohn's disease is chronic, possibly life-threatening, whereas a *C-diff.* infection can be cured . . . I think. But now, I'm distracted by a man in the next bed, a curtain separating us. He moans every fifteen seconds as if on schedule. A nurse is telling him he probably has diverticulitis.

"What's that?" he asks her.

"Usually a bit of nut or seed gets trapped in the intestine," she answers. "We need to run a CAT scan."

I try to remember the last time *I* ate a nut or a seed. Yes! I *did* eat canned nuts about a week or so ago. I want to make sure I don't have diverticulitis. I want the doctor to order a CAT scan for *me*—a full-body X-ray. But then I remember the

X-ray of Quizzle's lungs, pinpoints of white, multiplying spots. The vet carefully reviewed all her symptoms. At the time, I told the vet that I wished she were *my* doctor. She spent more time with Quizzle than any doctor ever spent with me, and was gentle, patient, smart.

"The tests are negative for *C-diff.*," Dr. Harkness says. But he adds that I should continue taking that *second* antibiotic to counteract the effects of the *first* antibiotic, clindamycin, just in case. That's all he can do. "There's no way to know for sure without a colonoscopy," he says.

"Then why can't I have one?" I ask.

"The gastroenterologist wouldn't order one yet. You have to wait and see if the metronidazole takes effect."

"You can't order it?" I ask.

"There's a procedure to be followed."

Community Hospital, November 3

People in good health usually don't get *C. difficile* disease. People who have other illnesses or conditions requiring prolonged use of antibiotics and the elderly are at greater risk of acquiring this disease. The bacteria are found in the feces. People can become infected if they touch items or surfaces that are contaminated with feces and then touch their mouths or mucous membranes. Healthcare workers can spread the bacteria to other patients or contaminate surfaces through hand contact.

—CDC

I awake with blurred vision. I stare at a line of text on my computer. Each letter possesses a shadow. I try another pair of reading glasses. The shadowed letters remain. *I am going blind.* Frightened, I return to the hospital, to learn that I'm only severely dehydrated.

"Please, can't you order a colonoscopy?" I plead from the bed where I'm again hooked up to an IV. Dr. Harkness is once again on ER duty. "Can't *you* do it?"

He shakes his head. "I'm not a gastroenterologist."

"Then could *I* call the doctor, schedule an appointment myself?"

"He wouldn't see you. The order has to come from me or Dr. Fields. It's still too soon. You have to wait."

Wait. For what? What he must mean, I think, is that I'm not sick enough, not frail enough, not emaciated enough. Why can't he see I need help *now*?

The County Hospital, November 23

If you are infected you can spread the disease to others. However, only people that are hospitalized or on antibiotics are likely to become ill. For safety precautions you may do the following to reduce the chance of spread to others: wash hands with soap and water, especially after using the restroom and before eating; clean surfaces in bathrooms, kitchens and other areas on a regular basis with household detergent/disinfectants.

—CDC

Marc drops me off at what we think is the emergency room as he drives off to park the car. It's not the right entrance, however. Through slushy snow and bitter wind, I wander down the street, around the corner. After feeling better for close to ten days, able to eat small doses of food—convinced the *C-diff.* infection, or whatever it was, is cured—I awoke this morning with a temperature and severe bouts of diarrhea. Of course, I'm unable to schedule an appointment with Dr. Fields this day before Thanksgiving. When I spoke by phone with her earlier, she suggested I go to the County Hospital in Muskegon, about twenty minutes away, a hospital with better diagnostic services than Community Hospital. She returned the emergency page from her home, pots and pans clanking in the background. Small pellets of anger pinged behind my eyes, although I'd never let her know. Sick, I have lost control of my body; I am entirely dependent on her.

Who is she?

I know nothing about her, not even where she attended medical school. After my previous doctor retired, I sought out Dr. Fields simply because she was a woman practicing at an all-women's clinic. I was sure that a woman doctor would be more nurturing, empathetic, understanding of my concerns. Is this lack of research on my part as irresponsible as not reading the warning labels on medication?

Today, on the phone, Dr. Fields told me to take aspirin for fever, Imodium for diarrhea.

I'd read on the Internet that it was harmful to take Imodium, that it encourages *C-diff.* to bloom. But what do I know? I'm too scared and weak to think straight. I took an aspirin. I swallowed an Imodium caplet.

I'm a good patient.

The clerk who admits me at the County Hospital is not interested in the fact that this is my fourth trip to an emergency room or that this mysterious infection vanished before recurring. *Just the symptoms, ma'am.* She writes up her form and points me down a corridor through a set of double doors that magically opens, as if I'm entering hell or Xanadu. Maybe both. By now, Marc has parked the car and caught up with me. We enter my curtained ER cubicle. I curl up under the covers, Marc on a plastic chair beside me.

"I'm Dr. Jones." A friendly young man in a white lab coat pulls back the curtain. "What seems to be the trouble?"

I give him the blow-by-blow with as many lurid details as I can remember. I make it sound as bad as possible. I want the works: every high-tech test performed *now*. I will refuse to leave the hospital without a diagnosis, a cure.

"We'll run some blood tests," he says, upbeat. "And a CAT scan, just to make sure."

A CAT scan! I'm thrilled. I want this superhuman machine peering beneath layers of skin, muscle, tissue, bone, into the core of every organ. Is my kidney acting as a kidney? liver, a liver? stomach? intestines? pancreas? bladder? I barely know what else gently throbs beneath my skin's surface. I don't understand the purpose of a pancreas, I realize. I don't question my body. Who wants to know how a body functions? To visualize the inner workings is horrifying. I just assume that every part knows its job and performs dutifully in order to keep this organism known as "me" functioning.

But who am I, really? I always imagined myself in terms of my mind, what I think, as well as how I appear, on the outside. I have reddish hair and hazel eyes. I'm five feet, three inches. Before I got sick, I weighed about 120 pounds. I'm a liberal Democrat. I vote in every election. I teach. Isn't *this* me? Who wants to know more?

But this doctor could care less how I voted in the last election. He wants to know when I last went to the bathroom, what I ate for dinner. "Does this hurt?" He probes my stomach. "This?" So now, wheeled into a giant doughnut of a CAT-scan machine, I imagine "me," who I am, differently. All of who I am is simply contained in a sack of skin. Without this body in some semblance of working order, does the rest of me matter?

This isn't my first CAT scan. About two years ago, a routine physical turned up blood in my urine. Three sonograms, one CAT scan, and a clean urine sample later, nothing was found to cause the abnormality. However, the CAT scan showed a speck of "something" on the lower tip of my lung. "It's probably nothing," the doctor said. "These new machines are overly sensitive." But just to be sure, the doctor ordered another CAT scan.

Nothing was found then.

Nothing is found now.

"The CAT scan is negative." Dr. Jones proudly smiles as if it's *his* body. "Everything looks perfect."

"So what *is* it, then?" I ask.

"Hepatitis A," he says, with confidence. "You have an elevated ALT level, and that's an indication of hep. A infection."

The nurse arrives with an IV, for fluids.

Dr. Fields's office, November 28

"Hepatitis A?" Dr. Fields exclaims. "Where would you have gotten that? Nothing points to that."

"A slightly elevated . . ." My voice trails off.

I spent Thanksgiving weekend thankful for the hepatitis A diagnosis, the least serious of the hepatitis alphabet—no active recovery regimen, just let it run its course. "In a few weeks, you'll be fine" were Dr. Jones's last words as they rolled me from the emergency room in a wheelchair.

Marc, who has driven me here to Dr. Fields's office, and I glance at each other and shrug. "I guess I picked it up somewhere," I say lamely, my euphoria flattening as yeastily as it'd risen only a few days before.

Dr. Fields appears stymied, not the look you want to see on your doctor's face. "How often have you gone to the bathroom today?" she asks.

"Twice."

"Well *that's* good," she says, wanting to cheer us up—since I probably went about twenty-three times over the endless Thanksgiving weekend.

"*But she's not eating,*" Marc says—Marc, who is usually shy and mild-mannered. "*That's* the only reason."

It's true: I've virtually stopped. I've lost more than ten pounds since October 30.

"Well, let's get her on an IV, then," Dr. Fields says. "Maybe now it's time to call Dr. Bright for a colonoscopy. A *C-diff.* infection or Crohn's disease wouldn't show up on a CAT scan."

My dehydrated skin is the texture of leather: black-and-blue bruised leather, from all the IVs. The nurse, searching for a vein, is unable to penetrate it with a needle.

After talking to Dr. Bright, the gastroenterologist, Dr. Fields orders me back to the County Hospital. Dr. Bright needs more lab tests before he'll perform the colonoscopy; maybe a nurse at the hospital will be able to hook me up to an IV.

The County Hospital, November 28

Although I'm not scheduled to stay the night, I'm assigned a room in the main wing. My roommate is a suicide survivor under a twenty-four-hour watch. It's not clear why the two of us are in a room together, given such dissimilar symptoms. Except that the very randomness, itself, is symptomatic. But symptomatic of what—like whatever disease I have—is difficult to say.

Now, since Dr. Bright needs more lab-test results, of course I'm unable to provide a stool sample. I'm dried out. Nothing is left. So they feed me anything I want. I realize I'm famished, starving. I devour a chicken-salad sandwich on gooey white bread, an oatmeal cookie, chicken noodle soup, and stewed prunes, which I've never eaten before. There's a good reason. They taste like syrupy dirt.

Pond water. Sludge at the bottom of a lake. Initially, all the food stays put in my system. The nurse suggests I walk around in order to speed things along. Up one corridor, down another. Marc accompanies me. Every room we pass is its own stage set or still-life of tragedy. I wonder what's wrong with all the patients; they probably wonder the same about me.

Later in the afternoon, Dr. Bright gets his specimen. After about a half dozen useless attempts, the nurse finally plunges an IV into my leathery skin. For four hours I watch the IV bag drip. I sense the suicide patient on the other side of the curtain; she rustles the sheets. Apparently she overdosed. They pumped her stomach. Maybe *this* is the connection: we've both evacuated our skin.

That evening, her young children visit, a boy and girl. The boy, breathless with drama, informs the nurse that *he* found his mother, called 911. The little girl pokes her head around the curtain to look at me. I stare back. We don't speak. I can't even smile, though I'd like to offer her encouragement to help her survive her mother. But who am I to speak?

On November 29 I receive the following e-mail from Dr. Bright's nurse:

colonoscopy and gastroscopy thurs. 12-1 at Community Hospital. register at 12:15. wednesday 11-30 clear liquid diet. wednesday at 5p. drink 1 and ½ oz. (3 tablespoons) of fleet phospho-soda mixed in 4 oz of water or ginger ale. throughout the evening you must drink at least 3 eight oz glasses of water or clear fruit juice. thursday at 7am drink 1 and ½ oz (3 tablespoons) of fleet phospho-soda mixed in 4oz of water or ginger ale. follow this with one glass of water or fruit juice. then nothing else by mouth until procedure. Fleet phospho-soda is available without a prescription. purchase 3 oz bottle. call if you have questions.

In order for Dr. Bright to perform the colonoscopy the next day, I must be spotless. The phospho-soda tastes like what I imagine nuclear waste would. With each swallow, I gag. My skin shivers sweat. Every ten minutes, or less, I am in the bathroom. By two in the morning, the black-and-white tiles on the bathroom floor seem to strobe. I don't feel the ground beneath my feet. I don't see my chest rise and fall with breath. I am all fluid, floating the nineteen steps between bedroom and bath. By six in the morning, I am polished stainless steel, scrubbed porcelain. My insides are scoured clean.

I am also desert-thirsty, pristine, parched. Each cell of my body rinsed with astringent, I feel light enough to float above the bed. The canary-yellow sheets waver like a flying carpet. Emptiness itself is a balm. It asks nothing of me, of my body.

I fantasize about lime popsicles.

Community Hospital, December 1

> *C. difficile* is generally treated for 10 days with antibiotics prescribed by your healthcare provider. The drugs are effective and appear to have few side-effects
>
> —CDC

Waiting for the colonoscopy, I lie under the covers of yet another hospital bed, now in the gastroenterology wing. As with previous visits to this hospital, my thin, freezing body is cocooned in a heated blanket; all their blankets are baked in stainless-steel stoves with glass windows. I ask for a new blanket whenever the warmth ebbs. Finally, I'm wheeled into the procedure area, where Dr. Bright waits for me. Yesterday, I typed a two-page, single-spaced outline of the entire saga to read to him: so I won't forget anything; so he'll have a full history, all possible relevant information. Patiently, he waits for me to finish the document.

"This time, we'll find out what it is," he promises.

"It's a *C. diff.* infection," he confirms, after I awake from the procedure with full-fledged, blessed amnesia. I remember nothing since the nurse initiated the anesthetic drip. He prescribes Vancocin, a *good* antibiotic, once again, to try to counteract the effects of the bad one, clindamycin. A ten-day supply of Vancocin, twenty-eight pills, 125 mg each, costs $370. One every four hours, a rigid schedule. Who knows what chaos will erupt if I miss a dose? 6 p.m. 10 p.m. 2 a.m. 6 a.m. 10 a.m. 2 p.m. I set the alarm. I stay on schedule.

On December 2, the day after the colonoscopy, Marc buys a copy of the

New York Times that has an Associated Press article headlined: "Deadly Germ Is Becoming Wider Threat." The item, datelined Atlanta, the headquarters of the Centers for Disease Control, warns of *Clostridium difficile* commonly seen in people taking antibiotics. Last year, I learn, it caused one hundred deaths in eighteen months in a hospital in Quebec. Now, according to the CDC, four states (Pennsylvania, New Jersey, Ohio, and New Hampshire) show the same bacteria in healthy people who have *not* been admitted to hospitals, or even taken antibiotics. The bacteria, now resistant to certain antibiotics, work against colon bacteria. Therefore, when patients take certain antibiotics, particularly clindamycin, "competing bacteria die off and *C. difficile* multiplies exponentially." The CDC report focuses on thirty-three cases reported since 2003. Of these cases, one woman, fourteen weeks pregnant with twins, lost the fetuses and died. The woman had been treated three months earlier with trimethoprim-sulfamethoxazole, for a urinary tract infection. Ten others among the thirty-three had taken clindamycin. However, eight of the thirty-three cases had not taken antibiotics within three months of the onset of symptoms. According to Dr. L. Clifford McDonald, an epidemiologist at the CDC, it's unclear what has caused this outbreak of *C-diff.* "In general," he cautioned, "if you have severe diarrhea, seek attention from a physician."

Marc buys a package of natural-fruit popsicles. I lie in bed, under the quilt, sucking on one. It melts on my tongue. I swallow. But it doesn't taste as good as I imagined the night before the colonoscopy. It's not what I want.

Days remain seamless, one dissolving into another, one Turner Classic Movie into the next. Hours revolve around these black-and-white images as well as the Vancocin cycle. Severe symptoms subside, though my insides feel chafed. When I wash my face, for example, it hurts to lean against the sink. My stomach feels as if it will explode. Or implode. I hardly know which. Rather than constant physical pain, however, I experience discomfort; or, more than discomfort, I fear my body will never again be normal . . . that the word "normal" will morph into new definitions. For now, "normal" remains a stomach that continues to rebel. My skin feels dry, transparent. Not enough moisture even to sweat. My hair hangs brittle, bone dry. My lips and knuckles are raw, chapped.

• • •

After the colonoscopy, I don't hear from Dr. Fields. She doesn't call to ask how I'm doing. I'm not surprised. I find a new doctor who orders my files from Dr. Fields's office. He tells me that the original lab tests came back normal: I never had a vaginal infection.

I write to Dr. Fields. I must be sure she knows about her erroneous diagnosis, as well as about the potentially deadly prescription. "I want to make sure that you never prescribe this antibiotic to any of your other patients. After spending about ten minutes on the Internet it was clear, even to me, that clindamycin should *only be prescribed in a severe medical emergency.*"

Health insurance covers most of the costs, but the final tally tops $11,000.

Six months after the first symptoms, I still have periodic discomfort and have regained only five pounds of the twenty I lost.

And while I never discover the cause of that ghostly fluttering pain in my abdomen—the reason for my initial appointment with Dr. Fields—it never returns. If it does, I will not attempt to shoo it away. Perhaps I will even welcome and bless it as a signal from beyond, a sign of my heightened appreciation for my body, or at least as a reminder that things could be worse.

Dr. Fields never responds to my letter. Instead, I receive a bill from her office for $260.

Sue William Silverman's first memoir, *Because I Remember Terror, Father, I Remember You* (University of Georgia Press), won the Association of Writers and Writing Programs award series in Creative Nonfiction. She is also the author of a second memoir, *Love Sick: One Woman's Journey through Sexual Addiction* (W. W. Norton), and a poetry collection, *Hieroglyphics in Neon* (Orchises Press). She teaches in the low-residency MFA in Writing program at Vermont College.

Keeping Up Appearances

Leslie Einhaus

Jajo, my maternal grandmother, never went anywhere without Juicy Red lipstick. She applied it upon waking, after coffee, between meals, and at bedtime. Jajo even awakened in the night to freshen her lips on quick trips to the bathroom—just a spot of color, in the event that Pop, my grandfather, woke up and saw her visage in the strands of moonlight sifting through the window of their double-wide. Along with the lip color, Jajo wore matching nail polish, Emeraude perfume, and cheap stilettos. She coiffed her red locks even for a shopping trip to the local five-and-dime. I recall once seeing my grandmother without her creams, foundations, eye spackle, lip color, and spritzes of hairspray when I was five or six. I shuddered. She seemed to me another person, standing there in her bra and panties, the scent of Emeraude almost choking me. "I need to reapply my face," she said, holding a cup of coffee, lipstick stains around the rim.

In Texas, the ritual of "putting on one's face" is passed from one generation to the next, along with recipes and family stories. From my mother's side of the family, I was given gifts of makeup from an early age and taught how to use it. Being perfect, or at least giving the impression of perfection, was important.

Things were a little different on my dad's side of the family. My other grandmother was a no-nonsense woman—no glittery baubles or sexy, open-toed shoes for her. Only on special occasions and with a little prodding would Grandma sweep the cosmetic blush across her sensitive skin. She would add just a hint of lip color—Autumn Gleam or Georgia Peach—for Saturday evening Mass, when she dipped her unpainted fingers into the bath of holy water.

Families, of course, are not perfect. My father grew up west of Dallas, Texas, in what is now the large metropolis of Arlington, where he lived with his parents, one brother, and five sisters. They've managed to help each other through divorces, alcohol abuse, grief, money challenges, and the plight of teenage pregnancy.

Each member of the family had difficulties and challenges; my grandfather, father, and aunt were linked by an inherited disease, rarely spoken about, and then only in whispers. Dad and his sister, Susie, more than ten years apart in age, were close because of their similar personalities, yet the disease brought them even closer, like a tightening of thread. The body is marked in psychological and physical ways by this disease, which leaves its sufferers far from perfect.

It is known as neurofibromatosis (NF), a primarily genetic disorder that causes tumors to grow along nerve pathways in the body. Tumors can appear on the body's exterior, a dozen to hundreds at a time, on the face, trunk, and legs. The tumors also can grow on the body's interior, hidden away; it might seem as though nothing is wrong, but the symptoms ignite like tiny flames, one after the other, until an entire portion of the body is overwhelmed by pain deep within.

NF1, the type of neurofibromatosis that runs in my family, is the most common form of the disease, affecting 1 in every 3,500 births around the world. It was once commonly believed that neurofibromatosis was the disease in *The Elephant Man* that horrified audience members. It's also been called "the whispering disease" because no one—physicians, patients, and family members—wanted to talk about it. That was certainly true in my family.

I don't recall the family's disease ever seeping into conversations I heard as a child. I recall very few references to tumors or surgery schedules, and never a mention of the name of the disease. It wasn't until high school, when I was diagnosed, that I found out about the intricacies of the disease. I am told now that the idea was to "get through it and move on."

Having any genetic disorder feels shameful. The word *disorder* itself conjures shameful, bone-chilling thoughts—it is all about you, your bloodline, and your inheritance. Having a disease like NF makes a patient feel vulnerable, not only physically but emotionally as well. Any appearance of perfection is shattered—something difficult for anyone to accept, but especially in a family like mine, which valued physical perfection.

Like my dad, I've had multiple surgeries within a few months. Each surgery brings new scars. These scars become a reminder of the disease, the amount of pain endured. They can cover the body like a giant connect-the-dots game, and though they may fade in time, they never completely vanish.

I remember one December, Dad being rushed to a hospital in Arlington from Grandma's house because of back pain caused by a slipped disk in his vertebrae. His yells erupted in the air like tiny volcanoes, so fiery hot the exclamations brought tears to my eyes. In what I remember as an expansive room with high ceilings and no windows for escape, the noise grew with such intensity that it eventually filled the room. My emotion spilled forth, the worry mounting as the minutes passed on my faded cartoon wristwatch.

I am told that Aunt Susie and Dad dealt with NF1 on a regular basis with surgeries every few years, when the pain became too intense. The gravity of the situation wasn't presented to me then, however. All I knew was that a tumor could press against nerve endings and cause jarring pain that eventually made surgery a necessity, and then Dad would go to the hospital. The reality of it hit me hard when I was in third or fourth grade and I overheard a conversation between my parents.

I've always remembered this scene with me sitting against the trunk of a tree, bone and skin against tree bark in the yard alongside the white farmhouse with the deep front porch I used as a stage. On a trademark sunny, humid Texas afternoon, I am next to an open window and I can hear the voices of my parents discussing the testing procedure, the possible results. Then again, maybe I was in the front room of the house that led out to the stage. I perk my ears toward the kitchen, a few steps away, where my parents are talking about the possibility of testing, a blood draw, what-if, and results via telephone. From the beginning, my parents seem in agreement that testing is off-limits.

"Why put her through that?"

"Even if she does have it, symptoms might not show up for years."

"If she gets it, she gets it. Why do we need a test to tell us?"

"I want her to live her life without all that fear."

My face reddens as I realize the "she" is me. I want some juice or a sip of water. I wonder if the test they speak of involves needles. I hate needles. I want to know I won't have surgeries and long hospital stays like Dad. Still, at this point,

I am unaware of what exactly the disease is and how it may affect me, if I am diagnosed.

"Remember, even if she has it, she may have no symptoms or very few."

"That's true."

"Look at you and Susie," Mom remarks. "You have surgeries here and there, but you still live your lives."

"All I know is that I don't want her to suffer. I'd take the pain on myself if I knew she wouldn't have it."

"Whatever happens, we can deal with it. Let's just see how things progress. She has no symptoms to speak of. Why even put it in her head?"

"Let Jimmy take his boys to get tested."

Jimmy did have his sons tested. Neither cousin inherited NF1. In the wake of the results, my parents stuck with their decision not to have me tested.

Dad always seemed to be exercising—running, walking the hunting dogs, or lifting weights. Postsurgery, he always seemed to recover quickly, with few complications. Watching him, I thought having the disease didn't seem like much of a burden. I didn't know about his inner turmoil and fears and serious symptoms that were kept secret from family, friends, and even medical professionals.

When I was diagnosed as a senior in high school, I remember Dad telling me I had to be strong. Then he told me he was sorry.

Yet, my suspicions had begun even earlier. I realized something might be wrong in fifth grade. I thought I might have cracked my tailbone after slipping on some ice. The bruised tailbone never felt quite right after that. When the tailbone pain didn't go away completely, I began to worry I might have what Dad had. The pain began to radiate down my legs, with the pain quotient rising like a thermometer's mercury during summers in Texas.

I didn't know a lot about what Dad had, but I did know it was hereditary. The tailbone injury stands out because it became, for me, the moment when the pain became a possible symptom. It became a warning signal that I might have this disease. The pain in my tailbone may have come from a slip on ice or, what I feared, from a growing mass that rested on a set of nerves.

Two years later, the injury came to the forefront again when I wanted to go sledding before our big Thanksgiving feast, up in Idaho at a condo we rented there. I was insulated from the cold on that overcast November day when I ignored my mother's worry and went sledding on a bumpy hill near our home. I tromped through the snow to the top where all my hesitation dissipated and I eagerly anticipated the exhilarating rush on slick, packed ice. I recall the snowflakes that fell on my puffy pink winter jacket. I dusted off the accumulation of snow, sat on the plastic saucer, and pushed off, snow clinging to my coat, pants, cheeks, and fleece snowcap. I continued sledding until dusk, ignoring warning prickles of pain.

That winter and spring, the pain came and went in my lower back and tailbone area, no matter what activities I chose. With the passing months, the sensation became deeper in my body, the pain sharper than any injury I could have sustained on ice. I knew something was wrong. The nerve "zaps," as I called them, jolted my entire body sometimes just as I was about to fall into deep sleep. Nothing, not exercises or pain relievers, could lessen the force that invaded my body.

But I never told a teacher, the school nurse, or even my friends. I never wanted attention, and I knew they would not be able to help me.

For the next several years, the pain continued off and on, varying in frequency and intensity until my senior year of high school, when I was unable to sit in a chair for any extended period. When two, four, or six extra-strength Tylenol didn't ease the pain, my private worry began to mount. Finally, I couldn't hide it anymore. As frightened as I was about the medical procedures, surgeries, and whatever else was ahead of me, I was more afraid of what might be wrong. My body was trying to tell me something. I could no longer be silent.

After a lengthy MRI scan at the local hospital, a neurosurgeon told me I had a tumor along my spine and one in my pelvis.

"The one in your pelvis looks questionable. There's a possibility it could be cancerous, though that would be unusual. But then again, there's always that chance," said Dr. Hill in his signature monotone. Wearing his starched white jacket and name-brand hiking boots laced in tight knots, he said, "We'll need to perform surgery soon."

I was left in the tiny exam room with Mom and a nurse. The room, void of color, filled with silence.

In the reception area, tears fell down my face. I looked out the window at the gray Ford pickup truck with Dad behind the wheel, waiting for the news.

Dad didn't like doctors. He also didn't want me to suffer, so his way of dealing with the situation was to remain on the outskirts, in the parking lot of the doctor's office, in his truck, waiting for the news he didn't want to hear.

Individuals with NF1 have a 50-50 chance of giving the disease to their children. Dad didn't want to know he had passed this dreaded disease to his only child. He just said the exam room was too small for the three of us. So Dad read magazines about wilderness preservation and how to take the best photographs of wildlife. He brought along coffee in a stained plastic mug. The truck's ignition roared to life before Mom opened the passenger door and let me in the backseat.

I take after my father in many ways: same long, oval face; thick, wavy hair; long, slender legs; and big, extra-narrow flat feet. But my skin is pale and dotted with freckles across the ridge of my nose, arms, and shoulders, and it burns when exposed to sun. A spritz of perfume applied directly to my skin can make it turn red.

Dad's skin was always darker than mine, a trait I envied because it hid his scars, especially the one at his neck. Dad worked at darkening his skin, though. He sat in front of the sunlamp to rid himself of any blemishes or "spots," as he called them—any imperfection.

Before he turned on the sunlamp in his at-home office and pulled the goggles around his thick dark brown hair, he gave me explicit instructions: "Don't come in here. Don't look at the light."

I was also like my dad in dealing with pain. I ignored it as best I could, though it wasn't always easy. Our strength in dealing with the pain associated with NF became, in many ways, our greatest weakness. Many times I glanced at Dad either in a hospital bed or perched in a wheelchair going home after surgery, and I wondered to myself, how did we get here? He never talked about the pain in a way that made for an understandable progression of events. Often, events seemed to be out of order or zooming along in fast-forward. He put up with his pain in silence until it got so bad he couldn't take it anymore and we rushed him to the emergency room. Other times, he scheduled a visit to the doctor's office alone, telling Mom and me only afterward.

Even before my own diagnosis, I noticed when Dad grabbed his lower back during chores around the house or when we went on weekend walks. He winced, bent over, his left palm against his lumbar region, and without even thinking I'd start a tiny prayer—*let him be OK.*

"My back just got caught." Dad would pull himself upright, struggling to smile.

"You're sure you're OK, Dad?" I would ask, looking into his face.

"I'm fine. It's OK."

Maybe sometimes it was, and maybe sometimes it wasn't. I look back and wonder. I desperately wanted everything to be OK, so I tried to believe him. In most cases, he brushed off the pain like most people dusted off snow.

After I was diagnosed, I knew how intense the physical pain could be. I also knew that whatever happened to Dad, in or outside a hospital room or surgical ward, could happen to me.

For a long time, I stayed silent. I didn't have a group of close friends in high school I could trust, and I didn't want people to know. If people found out at school, I worried they might make fun of me. My self-esteem wasn't terribly high, and being diagnosed with a disease didn't help. I worried about myself and about Dad in silence. At the time, I didn't know anyone else with a disease like ours, so it felt alien. No one could understand how we felt.

At home, the rule was: don't dwell on it. Live your life like you don't have anything wrong.

On countless occasions to relieve pain, I'd try stretching, pressing my hands into my lower back, thumbs against skin, nearly bruising myself. I would do almost anything to rid my body of pain.

"Go do some exercises—how about some squats, bend your knees, and stretch your back. That always helps me," Dad would say.

"It does help him," Mom chimed in.

So, I did what an only child does. I obeyed.

I bent my leg, stretched my back, my hands grasping my desk chair in my bedroom, my heels pointed toward the double bed. I stared up at a quotation on my wall about character and strength from Ralph Waldo Emerson: "Unless you try to do something beyond what you have already mastered, you will never grow."

But the pain persisted. The exercises never dissolved the pain, just masked it, providing only a brief reprieve. The pain always returned.

At least other people couldn't see the pain, like they could see the scars. By the time I graduated from college, I'd had multiple surgeries. A scar on my right shoulder that ran from across my collarbone to my bicep resembled the juiciness of medium-rare steak. Alone, I stared at it. Then, my eyes moved below my belly button to another scar, wider and longer, its color intense against my pale skin. Ugly. It curved toward my pelvis, resembling one of those lines on the topography maps Dad memorized for his hikes, only the line on my body was fatter and the color of some cosmetic blush. I was ashamed of the scars. "What's that?" a male friend of mine pointed to my right shoulder. "Looks like something gotcha there."

"Umm . . . ," I stammered, trying to decide what to say. I usually gave a response veiled in humor.

"I got attacked by a wild animal."

"No way, come on!"

"Surgical scar, actually."

"Wow. When did that happen?"

Sometimes I'd feel like answering; other times, I wanted to stop the inquiries. If someone seemed genuinely interested, I provided a detail or two.

In an effort not to draw attention to myself, I covered up the scars on my shoulders and back. I almost always opted for a dark-colored T-shirt with a collar instead of spaghetti straps or a tank top.

Sometimes, I'd stare at my body in the mirror and be overcome with emotion. I retreated under the patchwork comforter Mom made years before from leftover scraps of material—roses, Superman in flight, and solid squares the color of a moonlit sky. The yarn that tied it all together was the color of cotton candy. I stayed in bed, my cotton sheets and the comforter a canopy, and my tears, I noticed, smelled like rain.

In those moments wrapped in the covers, I'd worry whether someone would ever find me attractive. Would someone love me despite these hideous scars across my body, their numbers multiplying with each passing decade?

I was different from Aunt Susie, who lived her life with zeal. She carried her beer around on Christmas Eve, singing folksongs instead of traditional carols, her parents' living room filled with her friends.

Growing up, she never concentrated on NF1. She lived as though the disease never occurred to her. She lived without shame, with little worry about what others thought. Susie enjoyed lying out in the sun; she never let scars on her back and stomach stop her from wearing a bikini. I can see her petite frame strung across a metal folding chair or sprawled out on a towel in the sand, the straps and the scars intersecting at various angles, nearly indistinguishable.

I often visited her during trips to Arlington with my parents. I recall one visit on a long Easter weekend, when she was recovering from a surgery. Mom had volunteered to look after her that weekend. At the kitchen table, we dunked hard-boiled eggs into the paper cups filled with blue, red, and yellow dye from those kits you buy at the store. We set a colorful array of eggs on the back of the box with its perforated ovals. I recall our closeness then and how joy lit up her face. She had a personality like Dad's—light-hearted, funny, entertaining, and kind. After we decorated the eggs, we visited a nearby Catholic church that had organized a reading of the Stations of the Cross, which outlines the last hours of Jesus' life leading to the resurrection.

Susie and I never talked about the disease or what it was like for her. Mom tells me many stories about my aunt as a high school student in Arlington, a Kalamazoo co-ed, and a young bride. Even now, years after her death, I am inspired by how she approached life and by how much people enjoyed her presence.

When she was twenty-three, a cancerous tumor was found in Susie's pelvis and was quickly taken out. She underwent chemotherapy and lived five more years before the cancer returned. It is my understanding that tumors tend to hide away in areas like the pelvis, and have a higher chance of becoming malignant the longer they hide. In an act of prevention, I have yearly scans to keep track of any questionable lesions. If the surgeon feels they might turn malignant, they are removed.

Ignoring NF1 symptoms has the potential to kill you. At about the time I started high school and we moved to Idaho, Dad began to make a point of not keeping up with his symptoms and neglecting doctor visits. He wanted to spend time outdoors and with his family instead. He had occasional surgeries, but after a while he ignored the disease completely. He wasn't vigilant like he should have been.

A year after I graduated from college, Dad passed away from cancer. A tumor in his pelvis he waited too long to have checked became malignant and metastasized to his liver. Once the tumor was identified, it was too late. At first, doctors thought chemotherapy might be an option, but Dad didn't want to give up his time in the outdoors. He told the doctor he hiked on Tuesdays and Thursdays. Chemotherapy was a daily obligation. He didn't want to compromise.

From the day of the diagnosis, Dad lived just over a month—thirty-six days. He passed away at home with Mom and me and extended family present, including his mother. He was fifty-one.

In the months following my father's death, my scars began to signify something other than ugliness. They became something else entirely—signs of survival. I could live with this disease, if I kept on top of it. I had to be in tune with my body's workings. To falter significantly could mean death. A scar was just a scar. I began to find strength in these etchings on my skin. The scars reflect what I have gained through my experiences—as a patient and as a daughter.

I once had lunch with a friend from college, and she commented that I never complained about symptoms or surgery. "You hold it in so well," she said. At the time, I beamed with pride. Now, I don't see that as much of a compliment.

A few years after Dad's death, I was recovering from an NF-related surgery at my Mom's house in Lewiston, Idaho. I was already living independently, having taken a job at a nearby university. I was scheduled to recover for one more week before returning to my independent life.

One afternoon, when I was feeling particularly good, Mom and my Aunt Jamie, who was visiting from Texas, decided to take me shopping. They thought a trip to the mall and a makeover might boost my spirits. Jamie, my Mom's sister, had been taking care of me after my surgery while Mom taught school during the day.

When we entered the department store, I took in all the colors and textures of the clothes, eyed the shoes, and put earrings to my lobes. I was wearing navy sweats with no makeup, maybe a glide of clear gloss and a few blots of moisturizer. Despite my droopy cotton clothes, I felt invigorated just to be out in the world.

We went to the makeup counters, and I could imagine Jajo here, standing next to her two daughters in front of the stainless steel mirrors, wands thick with mascara placed inside slick navy blue cylinders perched at eye level. Tubes of used lipstick lined the slanted countertop. The image of lips puckered near glass, so close as to leave marks, reminded me of many moments when Jajo was alive and we'd gone on shopping sprees. She held shopping bags like trophies, her golden ankle bracelet gleaming like a smile.

Now, in this brightly lit showroom, I imagined her recommending a sassy shade of lipstick like Maraschino Cherry or Valentine Rose, her brightly painted nails clicking against the glass display counter, pointing them out.

"I don't need any foundation," I said, and told them about a friend from college who doesn't wear any makeup and looks fabulous.

"But Leslie, she has porcelain skin," Mom said, making eye contact with me.

"You can't get away without foundation," Aunt Jamie agreed.

"Before too long wrinkles will start cropping up on your face. You don't want that," Mom chimed in.

"Let's just see what shade works best for you." Aunt Jamie steered me toward the cosmetic counter with its rows and rows of high-priced goods.

"We'll get one that doesn't look cakey. I promise. I'll even buy it for you as a get-well present," Mom said.

I'd spent the past few weeks swallowing an assortment of pills and bland food from the hospital, overcoming bouts of lightheadedness and nausea. I felt too weak to rebel. I decided to go ahead and let the makeup artist apply the high-end cream to my face, something Jajo did every day of her adult life. I pulled back the strawberry-tinted hair I had inherited from her and centered myself.

On the black cushioned seat, no longer level with the crowds of shoppers, I noticed the blazing glare, the spotlight with the multitude of mirrors that surrounded my face. I was uneasy, so I took a deep breath. The makeup artist dabbed a raspberry blush on my skin. It felt smooth, and from what I could see, it added more glow to my cheeks than I'd seen in days. I gazed at my jawline where the makeup artist had feathered in the foundation. I couldn't find that line of demarcation. If only for that moment, my skin was, in fact, seamless.

Leslie Einhaus is pursuing an MFA in creative writing at the University of Idaho. She also is employed as a writer/editor in the university's Communications and Marketing Department. She lives in Moscow, Idaho, with her two Labradors, Bridger and Sierra.

Do No Harm

Pamela Lane

I hadn't looked into a mirror in a long time; I had no reason to see myself. I was not someone I wanted to know. But in his eyes I saw my reflection. In the horror and the disgust, I saw what he saw.

"My god, what happened to you?" The doctor stood just inside the exam room, exactly where he had pivoted after closing the narrow wooden door. He asked the question as if the answer would determine whether he would stay or leave.

I hesitated, confused, afraid. "I, ah, broke my jaw." He wore leather shoes. They stepped toward me. I felt him lift the sleeve of the cotton gown the nurse had given me. I tried to tell her it was just my jaw, but she insisted I take off my clothes and put on the gown. I had become a person who did not argue.

Every nine seconds in the United States a woman is assaulted and beaten. Four million women a year are assaulted by their partners. Every day, four women are murdered by boyfriends or husbands.[1]

My posture was so hunched that the gown fell open in the back. That had become my bearing, curled to protect my stomach and face, eyes down, invisible. I could feel him looking at me, even as I looked at my bare feet. He edged around me—moving the gown, prodding a little as he went—because the heavy exam table blocked him from circling. I sat on the end like when I was a kid on the edge of the diving board, waiting to jump in. I felt small like that, my bare feet dangling.

Domestic violence is most prevalent in women 16 to 24.[2]

• • •

"Who did this to you?" He touched my jaw for the first time, not hard, like the heavy steel of the .45 automatic that had left it dangling, knocked loose. I could still talk, which surprised me; I just wasn't sure what to say. So I lied.

"I fell."

"From the look of it, you've been 'falling' for a long time." He said "falling" in that sarcastic way popular kids use to be mean to the unpopular ones. He was right, though. It had been a long time, although I can't tell you how long, even now, looking back. Then, I had no time, I had nothing to mark time by.

He asked me who did it. I asked him for help. He kept asking, in that voice that said I was wasting his time. I told him I was afraid. I told him I couldn't tell him why. I remember crying. I remember the way he looked at me.

Treating battered women tended to evoke more negative emotional states than treating patients with infectious disease. Both [primary and nonprimary care physicians] exhibited negative feelings when confronting battered women.[3]

He walked to a phone hanging on the blue-green wall. The cord was tangled. He lifted the receiver. "I'm calling the sheriff."

I looked up into his eyes. "Please, please don't call the sheriff," I begged him.

I didn't tell him, but I had called the sheriff once. I told him I was being held in a farmhouse by a man who was going to kill me. He asked me how I knew the man. I said we had dated, but I had broken up with him. He'd said in his Texas drawl, "It sounds like a domestic dispute to me, little lady." He asked me how old I was, then told me I had a lot to learn about men. He said, "If he has a short fuse, you'd best learn not to make him mad." I told him about my family, how he planned to kill my little brothers and sister if I got away. The sheriff said maybe they could hold him overnight. Overnight. I hung up.

Victims of domestic violence are reluctant to report abuse. Women very reasonably fear retaliation.[4]

But that was not the only reason I didn't want the doctor to call the sheriff. Ken, the man who owned the pistol so clearly imprinted on my face, was a few steps away in the waiting room, high on cocaine, surrounded by women and kids waiting for immunizations or whatever people wait for in a small town doctor's office in rural Texas. He'd tried to get into the exam room with me, but the nurse in the small clinic refused. Before he went back to sit down, he squeezed my arm, looked at me, then glanced at the waiting room. I looked at them, the innocent ones, and knew what he meant. Before he agreed to take me to a doctor, he'd stuffed a knife as long as my forearm, in a leather sheath, into one ostrich-hide cowboy boot, the pistol that did this into the other, and another pistol into the back of his jeans, under his suede jacket. He had a flair for arming himself. He dropped extra clips into his pockets. He was not going to jail, even on the outside chance that any man in rural Texas in 1973 would think that he deserved to be there.

> In 2000, 1247 women were killed by an intimate partner . . . which accounted for 33.5 percent of the murders of women . . . Women are most likely to be killed when attempting to leave the abuser. In fact, they're at a 75% higher risk than those who stay.[5]

The phone made that off-the-hook beeping sound, which throbbed in rhythm with the pain in my head. But he didn't hang it up. "If you won't report the man who did this to you, I won't treat you." The doctor was angry, but not because I was a skinny twenty-year-old kid covered with bruises and burns and scabs, begging him to help me even though I couldn't tell him why I wouldn't talk to the sheriff. He was mad because I was wasting his valuable time. Because I wasn't worth that time. I wasn't worth helping. I don't remember what he said after "I won't treat you." Maybe he didn't say anything. I just remember how I felt. I don't know what I expected—I knew no one doctor could save me. I wasn't a fool, but walking in that clinic I had had hope: I was still a person. Walking back to my abuser, my jaw displaced, still in pain, denied basic human compassion, now I had no hope. That doctor confirmed what my abuser had told me over and over: I wasn't worth the air it took to keep me alive. I deserved what I got.

Many battered women experience social, institutional, and provider barriers to obtaining help from the healthcare system for . . . domestic violence.[6]

After that I stopped fighting back. I stayed with him because I could see no other place for me. I could never go back home to my family, whose lives I had put in danger by dating a madman. I couldn't go back to school, to friends, to the shadow of a life I did not deserve. I resigned myself to being whatever he told me I was—his girlfriend, his property, his whore.

I fantasized about suicide like some women fantasize about a trip to Paris—with longing. I never asked anyone for help again.

In 1998, 30,575 Americans took their own lives . . . The researchers found a strong connection between intimate partner violence and suicidal behavior.[7]

If there had been a "Least Likely to be Victimized" category in my high school yearbook, my picture would have been there, showing a blonde in a hippie dress with an SDS fist button prominently displayed on it. It is a fallacy that race factors into the battering of women, or that women from the middle and upper classes are immune to abuse. I was white, middle-class, and a liberated, self-aware, politically active tough cookie. I would never let a man hit me.

And I didn't, at first.

I met Ken through a girl I had known in high school. Amy and I hadn't been close friends, but she was a stoner and I was a radical, and in the 1960s that was enough to make us both outcasts—counterculture friends by default. I'd lost touch with her when I'd dropped out of high school and hitchhiked to Boulder, Colorado, when I was sixteen. After a year of working at an FM underground radio station and having adventures, I returned home to get my GED and attend an "alternative" college.

I had high hopes for college, and life in general, but the reality of working a crappy full-time job, paying 100 percent of the costs of school, living with parents who required me to babysit my younger siblings to earn my keep, and going to school nights and weekends was just mutilating my idealistic dreams of adulthood. I had failed to find another radio job, and being a seventeen-year-old high school dropout with a sketchy work history didn't qualify me for any fun job. This surprised me, although I now can't imagine why. I took a sales job in a boutique near the university. The pay was awful and the owner was, in my easily expressed opinion, a monster. I had been a poor, but cool, person of some stature in Boulder—but in Tucson, I was a loser. Responsibility sucked. Poverty sucked. Anonymity sucked.

And then Amy called. It was my twentieth birthday, and I didn't have a date, or enough friends or money to rate a party. She had the solution, and he would be there at seven to pick me up.

The moment I saw him at the door to my parents' house, I was uneasy. It wasn't his long hair, parted down the middle like those velvet pictures of Jesus, or even the cowboy boots, skintight Wrangler jeans, huge silver buckle, western-cut jacket, or felt cowboy hat in his hand. Although the combination of those things in 1972 seemed odd, it wasn't enough to dissuade a girl in a serious dating drought on her birthday. It was his eyes: deep-set, dark, evil. Pull-the-wings-off-doves, fol-low-you-around-the-room, scary eyes. I looked beyond him, at a huge black Pon-tiac with black-tinted windows and new dealer tags that hulked at the curb.

"Pam?"

"Yeah?"

"Ken Cummings, ma'am." He tilted his head as if he would have tilted his hat, like John Wayne, if it hadn't already been in his left hand. "Mighty pleased to meet you." He revealed a dozen yellow roses from behind his back. "Happy Birthday." He extended them toward me, and I opened the screen door.

Roses. No boy had ever brought me roses. Of course, he was no boy. He must have been near thirty. Amy had told me he was from Texas and that he was rich, although I assumed at the time that one meant the other—everyone from Texas was rich. He was in business with her boyfriend, her "old man." I knew what kind of business—the only kind that brought men like this to a border town like Tuc-son: dope. I didn't care, though. He was supposed to take me to a fancy restaurant, and it was just one night. What could happen?

I'd never been to such an expensive place. On the way we'd smoked a joint while listening to quadraphonic sound in his cushy, velvet upholstery, so I was starving. He ordered for me. I didn't think anything of it, since I wouldn't have ordered the most expensive things, and he did, so happy birthday to me. He lit my cigarettes with a gold lighter and opened the doors—even of the car door, though he had to kinda jog around to beat me to it—and he almost wrestled the waiter to pull my chair out for me. I knew enlightened women didn't allow such nonsense, but he was from Texas, and being liberated wasn't getting me anywhere lately.

I ordered a slo gin fizz, even though I didn't drink, because I thought it made me look more grown-up and sophisticated; and even though I was underage, the waiter never asked me for ID. Ken called me "ma'am" all night, which seemed kinda creepy, and after dinner he opened a little amber glass bottle and offered me cocaine. Cocaine, rich man's speed. Everyone knew that it wasn't addictive, so I said OK. I liked it. I liked everything about the night—except for him. He gave me the willies.

He talked some about Texas and a lot about Vietnam. He really hated "gooks," as he called them, but I felt sorry for him, being sent to that unjust war and not knowing the true nature of the conflict. I explained it to him, because that's what I do: I explain things so people can see how misguided they are, especially about politics. He nodded like a bobble head, like he wanted me to shut up but was too polite to tell me.

I waited for his hand to stray "accidentally" onto my exposed leg or around my shoulders, but it didn't happen. I prepared an excuse for not wanting to go to his apartment, but he never asked. He didn't try anything. He just jogged around the car in front of my parents' house to beat me to that door handle—although by then I knew I was supposed to wait. I didn't want to put him into goodnight kiss territory as I squeezed by him to get out the car door, but he didn't try for the kiss. He just took off his hat and thanked me. I beat it to the front door and vowed never to see that freak again. But by the next weekend, after I'd ignored a couple of his calls, I couldn't remember exactly why I shouldn't go out with the rich guy who was so polite. He had so much, and I had so little. I deserved to be treated nice. And so it started.

Over the next few months, every time we went on a date it was the same: he took me to great places, got me high, never got fresh, and I ignored the voice in my head that said I should be afraid of this guy. The only thing that changed was that from the second date on, before I left him for the night, he would press a little amber bottle into my palm. My present. My payment.

Finally, one afternoon I went with him to a friend's house. Only it wasn't a friend. It was a Mexican dope dealer. They argued, Ken pulled a gun on him, and the world spun out of control. I wanted to get away, to go home. He took me to his apartment instead. That night was the first time he paraded his weapons, a pad-locked closet full of them, and told me the story of how he had fragged a young lieutenant in 'Nam and got away with it. He laughed. He acted out the scene with a machine gun–looking weapon that I no longer recall the name of. He hated greenhorn officers telling him what to do. The second time he killed one, they sent him stateside, to a military hospital in Corpus Christi for a few weeks, then they gave him a medical discharge. He was too dangerous to go back to Vietnam, but not too crazy to be released into the general population. He was ready for his new life, although he missed killing gooks. "Semper Fi, motherfucker."

I told him I didn't feel well, that I needed to go home. He hit me hard enough to knock me down. Then he raped me on the floor. I fought him until he got that rifle against my neck, his weight bearing down on each end of it. I needed both hands to keep it from crushing my windpipe, and even then I couldn't get enough air to struggle. I can't remember the details after that. I just know from the bruises and where I was sore that he did a lot more to me than I can remember.

When it was over he cried like a child. He let me leave the next morning, pretending I was only going to school. I wasn't about to call the police on a drug dealer—that was a death warrant. So I called Amy and told her what happened, told her to keep him away from me. She apologized profusely and agreed.

A few weeks later, she called and told me that Ken had ripped off the Mexican mafia for a kilo of cocaine, and they were looking for me because I had been with him at someone's house and he had identified me as his "old lady." She said she felt terrible because I would be hurt when they found me. She said she felt responsible, so she had an offer for me. She and her old man, who had also been ripped off by Ken and had to leave town, would pay me a thousand dollars to accompany her on a quick run to Houston. She and I would fly in for one day and fly right back. And I'd get enough money to go somewhere safe.

Her boyfriend was waiting with a car in Houston. I didn't even ask how he got there. I wasn't suspicious. As we drove away from the city, instead of into it, he had a rational explanation. So when we eventually pulled up to an old white farmhouse at the end of a very long dirt road, off of a series of narrow blacktop roads through the East Texas pine forest, I wasn't paying attention. It wasn't until we walked up the steps onto the porch and the door opened that I figured it out. Ken paid Amy and her boyfriend one pound of cocaine, approximately half of the stolen kilo, for me. I begged them not to leave me. On my knees, in tears, I begged them.

They never looked back.

I did eventually escape. By then my abuser had lost some of his violent fervor for me; I was no longer the pretty, self-confident, know-it-all he had abducted to punish for the crimes of all sinful women, but an overweight, compliant shell, deadened to all emotion—including fear. My abductor had stopped threatening to kill my family, and I didn't care if he killed me. He needed money and sent me to work. Ironically, the job I found was as a receptionist in a doctor's office. Ken took my paychecks, but he couldn't take what I was really getting from my job: confidence. The doctor, who knew about the abuse and avoided the subject, and the rest of the people I came into contact with at my job treated me with respect and dignity, and that reminded me what it was like to be a person. The doctor helped me with an advance on my salary and by cosigning for the utilities for an apartment, the location of which he and the staff agreed to keep secret.

> 50% of the homeless women and children in the U.S. are fleeing abuse. The amount spent to shelter animals is three times the amount spent to provide emergency shelter to women from domestic abuse situations.[8]

I left with what little I had, and shortly afterward my abuser abducted another woman, a cocaine customer of his, and her six-year-old child. She leapt from his car somewhere in New Mexico. Although she also knew her attacker prior to the abduction—and that had been the criterion quoted by the sheriff for not helping me—she was in her thirties, and from a prominent local family. I suspect no one told her it was only a "domestic dispute."

Ken went from jail to a forced thirty-day commitment in a VA lockdown, which turned into a near twenty-year series of incarcerations. But he was never punished for what he did to me.

I suffered for many years with debilitating headaches, asthma, colitis, allergies, paranoia, and vicious night terrors and was later diagnosed with post-traumatic stress disorder.

Women who are battered have more than twice the health care needs and costs than those who are never battered.[9]

Up to 64% of hospitalized female psychiatric patients have histories of being abused as adults.[10]

I was too ashamed to return to my family and had no money for, or understanding of, therapy. For years I self-medicated my depression, insomnia, and shame with drugs and alcohol.

Some years later, my best friend, who is a paraplegic, called to tell me that her boyfriend had beaten her up. She was at the emergency room, in her wheelchair, bleeding. He was at her house. By the time I got to her condo, a two-hour drive, I had acted out a hundred times in my head the scene that would take place. I had checked and triple-checked the weight in my pocket.

His car was out front. I silently thanked god. I don't know what I would have done if he'd left on his own, I was so pumped-up. When he answered the door, I walked in calmly. He never looked down to see what was in my hand until it was too late. I didn't want to kill him; I wanted to make him soil his pants. I wanted him to know what it felt like to be helpless, to fear for his life. And I did. With a pistol shoved up into the soft flesh under his jaw, I made him believe. He wept and begged me not to kill him. I made him promise to leave and never come back, told him that I would track him down and kill him if he did. I told myself I was doing it for her, but that was only partly true. I did it for me. And I didn't feel bad about it. She came home from the emergency room, and we got high and celebrated his exit from her life. I had saved her. I was a hero.

I had told this story dozens of times when it finally dawned on me: normal people don't stick loaded guns into other people's throats. I knew there was at least one gun in her house—what if he had called my bluff? What if he had overpowered me and shot me? What if I had shot him? There were many righteous responses to her situation that did not necessitate brutality—at least not by me.

I was not free of Ken just because my body was free; my submerged rage had a tripwire that was turning me into the twisted psychopath that had taken me by force all those years ago—right down to the pistol and the little amber bottles of cocaine.

I sought out treatment for my addiction and rehabilitation for my burned-out soul and was fortunate to find free, community-based therapy groups that allowed me to address the PTSD and its causes in a supportive manner. Almost all of my associated medical conditions resolved by themselves.

I haven't told the story of what I did to that man in over twenty years. I am no longer proud of it. I no longer own a gun.

In my second year of therapy I had been told to pay attention to how I was feeling—and without drugs it was hard to dodge those feelings. I realized that I always got depressed around my birthday—and I wasn't yet old enough for my inevitable decay to be the cause—so I started to practice the techniques the group leader taught us. I sat night after night and wrote in spiral notebooks, just stream-of-consciousness stuff: "I feel like crap. Life sucks. I don't know why I feel like crap . . ." Until it came out of my pen, the story of the doctor who turned me away, I didn't make the connection. I'd turned twenty-one unable to chew, subsisting on what I could get through a straw, in pain—the pain in my jaw and head, and the pain in my heart where hope had once been. That was my special birthday, the official beginning of womanhood.

Many women never get the help I got, and their low self-esteem traps them in the cycle of abuse and addiction—even if they escape the initial violence.

The silence was described as collusion between the abused women and other members of society: "The unspoken agreement between battered women and other members of society not to disclose or address the battering."[11]

The shame and silence that surrounds abuse fuels the problem. In spite of changing laws and education, the incidence of intimate partner violence (IPV) continues to increase. And women continue to suffer in silence, invisible to the rest of us. Since 1993, when the American Medical Association launched its land-mark "Campaign Against Family Violence," violence against women and girls has escalated. The free programs where I got help lost their funding and were closed.

My story was unique only because of the way I got there—not what happened to me when I was being battered. Now, with the education a person gets from watching TV, I would know that I could call the FBI. That taking a minor across state lines is a major crime, the kind of crime for which they hold a person for more than one night. My life was forever altered not just because a homicidal Vietnam vet targeted me, but because I could find no help, no hope, no reason to live.

It is caring health professionals who need to be the frontline of protection for battered women. It is not just women that suffer, but all of us. When the fabric of civilized society is rent, we all feel the split. In 2004 the *British Medical Journal* stated that "intimate partner violence is a major public health and human rights issue."

Sadly, protector of women is a role many doctors are loath to play. In a study of Australian general practitioner attitudes toward victims of domestic abuse, one rural female doctor expressed a common sentiment about the effective treatment of battered women:

> You often don't want to be too good at it because you get too many of them ...You might find people start referring them to you.[12]

If doctors ignore or humiliate patients who need help, and embrace the silence that is women's legacy in a society that blames them for their own abuse, battered women will continue to be injured and killed—and their children will perpetuate the victimhood and violence they have seen and often experienced.

Physicians need to understand their role in this cycle and practice the words of Hippocrates, the father of medicine, who admonished physicians to make a habit of two things: "to help, or at least do no harm."[13]

Pamela Lane is a freelance editor and writing coach and a writer/producer for television. She is a published poet at work on her first nonfiction book, a biography of Sharon Mitchell, PhD, entitled *Growing Up Naked in Public.*

1. Women's Rural Advocacy Programs (WRAP), "National Statistics about Domestic Abuse," http://www.letswrap.com/dvinfo/stats.htm.
2. C. J. Newton, "Domestic Violence: An Overview," *Find Counseling.com* (formerly TherapistFinder.net) *Mental Health Journal*, February 2001, http://www.findcounseling.com/journal/domestic-violence/.
3. S. Rabin et al., Israeli *Medical Association Journal* 2, no. 10 (2000): 753–57.
4. Newton, "Domestic Violence."
5. WRAP, National Statistics about Domestic Abuse.
6. M. A. Rodriguez, S. S. Quiroga, and H. M. Bauer, "Breaking the Silence," *Archives of Family Medicine* 5, no. 3 (1996): 153–58.
7. Centers for Disease Control, *Injury Fact Book*, http://www.cdc.gov/ncipc/fact_book/26_suicide.htm.
8. WRAP, National Statistics about Domestic Abuse.
9. National Organization for Women, "Violence against Women in the United States," www.now.org/violence/stats.html.
10. WRAP, National Statistics about Domestic Abuse.
11. Jeanne McCauley, MD, MPH, et al., "Inside Pandora's Box," *Journal of General Internal Medicine* 13 no. 8 (1998): 549–55.
12. A. Taft, D. Broom, and D. Legge, "General Practitioner Management of Intimate Partner Abuse," BMJ, doi:10.1136/bmj.38014.627535.OB (published 6 February 2004).
13. Hippocrates, *Of the Epidemics*, written in 400 B.C.E., translated by Francis Adams, http://classics.mit.edu.

In Praise of Osmosis

Jill Drumm

Critical care nurse Crystal Diggs can't help but think of Jell-O when she looks at her patient's chart. The kidneys of the patient in Room D210 are rebelling because they are trying to do the equivalent of sieving Jell-O through a coffee filter. But instead of cherry-red or lime-green gelatin, his kidneys are straining to filter myoglobins, large molecules released into the bloodstream when muscle fibers begin to break down—a process called rhabdomyolysis. The common course of treatment is a cycle of fluids and a diuretic, Lasix, but the patient's blood urea nitrogen (BUN) and creatinine levels have continued to rise, which means his kidneys are not filtering these protein-metabolizing by-products effectively, even with the Lasix treatment. If the levels don't stabilize and the rhabdomyolysis goes unchecked, his kidneys will be damaged irreversibly and he could die. Someone has to figure out what to do next. Whatever that is, it must happen soon.

Repeated blood work for Mr. Rhabdo indicates that the diuresis treatment still isn't working. Crystal knows that forced diuresis can also be harmful if continued when ineffective. She believes that the next step in his treatment should be continuous renal replacement therapy (CRRT). Unlike the intermittent or episodic forms of dialysis, CRRT takes over the patient's kidney functions for an uninterrupted period of time, and the metabolic waste products are removed from the bloodstream without straining the already damaged kidneys. The good news is, because the kidney's tubular cells regenerate, the damage can be temporary and sometimes can be resolved, with appropriate and timely treatment.

Selling the idea to Mrs. Rhabdo is a snap. She has only to look at her feverish husband hooked up to a ventilator, fluttering in and out of consciousness, to grasp the wisdom of a new treatment plan. He has developed a malignantly high fever in reaction to medication he was given during surgery, which resulted in the muscle damage that then caused rhabdomyolysis. Mrs. Rhabdo is also a nurse, employed at another hospital, and she looks too young to be the wife of a man so ravaged and worn-looking. None of her training has prepared her for this. She isn't a critical care specialist, so she's only generally acquainted with the continuous dialysis therapy that Crystal describes. But she knows enough to understand the danger her husband is in.

Crystal watches the two of them together, sensing the pain of that moment of white-hot realization that everyday life has been placed on a high shelf, out of reach. The husband and wife in that room are bound by a membrane forged out of the unspoken details of their "before" life. Our lives are shaped by small moments: the morning paper, a glass of wine before dinner, the cat crawling on your head at first light. During the hours she waits beside him, the wife wills the silence to be healing, like the busy silence of seeds gestating underground.

Crystal has been a wife. She knows that in this woman's place, she would focus on hope, a spark of momentum created by the sense of doing something to bring her husband back relatively whole, back to something like their routine "before" life. She'd choose that over waiting and over caution. Yes, Crystal decides, Mr. Rhabdo needs CRRT therapy immediately.

The unit where so many patients die or linger near death for weeks and months is womb-colored. Double doors grant access to the Trauma/Surgical Intensive Care Unit at this Tampa hospital. Walking into the unit, with its low ceilings, salmon-pink walls, red kidney bean–colored trim, cream and mauve tile floors, is like finding a sensory mute button. The colors, the quiet, the sanitized air—all of it as deliberately subdued as a holy space—cushion the healthy against their encounters with the critically ill.

If you ignore the locked drug cabinet, the large flat-screened monitor tracking patients' vital signs, the photocopied flyers posted outside every patient room advocating strict hygienic precautions—if you ignore those, the place seems like a typical office. In the hallways or nurses' station, staff members chat about the Tampa Bay Bucs game airing on a TV set in an unoccupied room. A torn, coverless phone book is left out on the counter. Stamped on the outer edges of the phone book pages like obscene graffiti is an attorney's ad in blue ink: *INJURED? Call 1-800-Ask-Dave.* A resident scoops up the last piece of pumpkin pie left on a small worktable before going back to his charts. The hub of the unit, the nurses' station bordered by hallways on three sides, is the point of entry between the living and the gravely sick. It's a clear threshold. It's also one the ICU nurses traverse easily, several dozen times over a twelve-hour shift. Inside a patient's room, nurses move efficiently among the machines, tubes, and wound dressings, clear in their mission of diligent care.

Patients here are the sickest anywhere. If you are gravely ill anywhere from Tallahassee to Naples, chances are excellent you'll wind up here, at one of the major trauma centers in a state of nearly 18 million residents. Nurses like Crystal Diggs, who spend twelve hours a day facing all the endless ways the human body can break down, make this ICU the place you would want to be if you were facing the possibility of death.

Crystal whisks across the hall to the nurses' station to phone the chief resident. She stares absently at a poster board cutout of a cornucopia and a turkey another nurse has taped on the patient's door, trying to figure out the best way to discuss her request with the chief resident, Dr. Gee. In her experience, straight to the point is best. She relates Mr. Rhabdo's latest lab results and her opinion about discontinuing the current course. Dr. Gee knows that Crystal is a "superuser," a highly trained specialist in CRRT. He agrees with her recommendation and asks her to consult with Dr. Eff, an attending nephrologist who could order the treatment.

This is part of a critical care nurse's job, the sometimes tricky negotiation of the hospital hierarchy. A primary attending physician usually has a team of primary care resident physicians working under his guidance, and a chief resident like Dr. Gee is highly regarded and experienced. In this case, there's also an attending nephrologist, Dr. Eff, who oversees the work of a nephrology fellow (similar to a resident), whom we'll call Dr. Fellow. Typically the residents and fellows have more interaction with patients and nurses than the attending physicians, though the latter are ultimately responsible for the decisions their residents or fellows make while under their supervision. Crystal must follow the consultation hierarchy among hospital physicians and request the CRRT treatment from Dr. Fellow.

She watches for Dr. Fellow's arrival as she checks on other patients. She doesn't know him well, and she wonders if he is the sort of doctor who tunes out any advice issued from the lips of nurses, despite their knowledge and experience.

Crystal often tells her own trainees, "If you keep trying to filter the Jell-O after the filter is clogged, eventually you will not be able to push any more Jell-O—or water—through the filter." Sensible food analogies work fine with trainees, but she isn't willing to bet that Jell-O will persuade a nephrologist. So she gets busy looking for the file she keeps of studies that support CRRT treatment in rhabdomyolysis patients. *Just in case,* she thinks, as she clips a copy of the statistics to the patient's chart. There's a chance the doctor will see this as anything but helpful—he might very well be annoyed because he perceives Crystal as being presumptuous or provocative—but it's a chance Crystal is willing to take. A bruised ego is nothing compared to what Mr. Rhabdo is facing.

Crystal is the conduit through which the team of doctors coordinates a patient's care. She speaks for patients and their loved ones, silenced by trauma and illnesses that can at times overwhelm even the most carefully structured systems.

Crystal knows Mr. Rhabdo is at risk of losing all kidney function, even dying, from acute tubular necrosis (ATN). The mortality rate in acute renal failure can run as high as 70 percent, depending on the underlying causes and the presence of other health problems. ATN is a common cause of kidney failure because it is a deterioration of the renal system's tubular cells, the microscopic pipes in the kidney's filtering apparatus. Tubular cells are normally in a continuous process of death and regeneration. When the cellular renewal cycle is interrupted by disease or injury, however, the system quickly goes into overload.

Crystal is convinced that this breakdown in Mr. Rhabdo's kidneys will eventually trigger a chain reaction in his body, leading to systemic failure. Without a change in treatment, he could drown internally.

When Dr. Fellow pauses to look over the charts in an alcove near the nurses' station, Crystal approaches him with the chief resident's orders for CRRT treatment.

He listens to her explanation and then decides. "There's no indication for what you want." He doesn't look up from what he's reading. Crystal is certain she has miscommunicated her request. The air-conditioning bailed a few months ago, and they are standing near the proxy air handler that sprouts white flexi-coil tubing and feeds air into the ceiling ductwork. Perhaps he hasn't heard her.

"But I have all of this research that does indicate this treatment. Right here." Crystal leans over his shoulder, pointing at some of the statistics she has highlighted. He shakes his head while she talks and shrugs his shoulder impatiently, like a horse flicking its tail at a fly.

Crystal repeats, "But the treatment *is* indicated."

Other nurses pause or slow down in their tasks, ears cocked in alert toward the intense exchange happening just outside Room D210. Over Dr. Fellow's shoulder, Crystal sees the patient's wife standing in the doorway of her husband's room. Her eyebrows are drawn up in disbelief. Crystal taps the report again, standing up to her full five-foot, one-inch height, and willing calm into her voice. It's hard for her to resist the reflex to adopt a "put up your dukes" stance when protecting someone under her care.

Dr. Fellow keeps writing in the patient's chart. Crystal lets a long silence pass, hoping he is reconsidering.

"We will not be starting dialysis," he repeats. "Period," he adds, slamming the chart shut. Crystal watches the back of his neck, noticing the scarlet flush of anger contrasting against his white coat collar as he walks away.

Mr. Rhabdo is a few minutes longer without the treatment Crystal is convinced he must have. In her mind's eye, she can see the coffee filter clogged with Jell-O.

As it turns out, Crystal's patient's condition is an apt metaphor for the problem many well-informed people believe is the number one threat to our health care system. It's also a strong analogy for the situation Crystal faced with Dr. Fellow in late 2004. Silence is a membrane. Its thickness, and thus its permeability, is dictated by the kinds of silence the medical community can unwittingly enforce: the silence of unassailable authority, the silence of fear, or the silence of "not my problem." Fortunately, as the demand for increased medical accountability (and the number of lawsuits against hospitals) has increased, that membrane is thinning, raising pressure to create change. In osmosis, water molecules move from areas of high concentration to low concentration through a semipermeable membrane, such as a cell wall. Effective communication is an isotonic state, where flow occurs in equal force in both directions through a semipermeable membrane. Balance—whether psychological or physiological—is good.

In 2005 an organizational-performance consulting company, Vital Smarts, released a report titled *Silence Kills: The Seven Crucial Conversations for Healthcare*, which soundly concluded that communication breakdown is at the root of most medical errors. Vital Smarts cofounders Kerry Patterson, Joseph Grenny, Ron McMillan, and Al Switzler authored two best-selling books, *Crucial Conversations: Tools for Talking When Stakes are High* (2002) and *Crucial Confrontations: Tools for Resolving Broken Promises, Violated Expectations, and Bad Behavior* (2005), that address communication problems in personal and professional situations. The firm's awareness of communication breakdown as a major culprit in medical errors has grown over the last two decades, as it has studied organizational behavior. After nearly twenty years of witnessing and analyzing problems within health care systems, Vital Smarts decided to quantify the issue through thorough research. One of the authors of the *Silence Kills* study, David Maxfield, describes the problem this way: "Hospitals are the epitome of a knowledge organization, where the name of the game is how to get the right information from the right person to the right person—at the right time and in the right form. Whenever that breaks down, health-care breaks down. Communication is the lifeblood of the healthcare process."

The observations of organizational behavior documented by Vital Smarts have proved over and over that "the most pervasive and pernicious problem that keeps other problems from being solved is people's inability to speak up about them," according to Grenny, coauthor of both the *Crucial* books and the *Silence Kills* study. Researchers interviewed over 1,700 nurses, doctors, and health care administrators and confirmed the systemic nature of communication pathologies in health care. The authors examined issues they feel are the most difficult and yet the most crucial for health care workers to safely and effectively address: broken rules, mistakes, lack of support, incompetence, poor teamwork, disrespect, and micromanagement. They concluded that 88 percent of doctors and 48 percent of nurses and other health care providers "work with people who show poor clinical judgment." Perhaps even more alarming: "Fewer than ten percent of physicians, nurses and other clinical staff directly confront their colleagues about their concerns, and one in five physicians said they have seen harm come to patients as a result." This study also found that the ability to hold crucial conversations—"emotionally and politically risky discussions"—is key to creating safety and accountability in the health care environment.

Silence Kills was released in conjunction with the *American Association of Critical-Care Nurses (AACN) Standards for Establishing and Sustaining Healthy Work Environments*, which is, in part, a call to action for increased communication skills. Vital Smarts also conducts two-day Crucial Conversations seminars for members of the more than 240 AACN chapters in the United States. The focus in improving health care is shifting to creating skilled communicators, because, according to the *Silence Kills* study, three in four medical errors are caused by mistakes in interpersonal communication. The study concludes that "with 195,000 people dying each year in U.S. hospitals because of medical mistakes, . . . creating a culture where healthcare workers speak up *before* problems occur is a vital part of the solution."

The AACN spent a year and a half studying health care environments and writing its own report on sustaining safe and healthy work environments, which addressed six issues: skilled communication, true collaboration, effective decision making, appropriate staffing, meaningful recognition, and authentic leadership. One of the directors of AACN, Dana Woods, says that these six issues are "seemingly simple, intuitive things that need to happen in the work environment, and we all know it, the same way we all know that if we exercise more and eat less, we're going to lose weight. But it's really hard to do." That they are simple and intuitive is perhaps the reason why, until the study and the AACN standards were released, communication and collaboration were considered "soft issues" or "soft skills."

Mr. Rhabdo is fortunate. He has a nurse who is not only a highly trained clinician but also a tenacious advocate of healthy communication.

When Dr. Eff, the attending nephrologist, appears on the unit later that day, Crystal again pulls out her folder of supporting research. "Here are Mr. Rhabdo's results. You can see that his kidney function is declining. Dr. Fellow didn't think so, but this patient needs CRRT." Crystal keeps the growing frustration out of her tone as she sees the doctor's expression shift into a frown. Research and diplomacy aren't enough to make her point.

"No," Dr. Eff says. That's all. He's confident the matter is closed. He scribbles his signature on the nephrology fellow's progress notes and leaves the unit without another word.

"It was like a brick wall," Crystal remembered later. "I just didn't understand."

Crystal had never met Dr. Eff before, which made trying to understand his refusal even more difficult. She would learn later that he wasn't one of the regular attending physicians, that he was covering for another nephrologist. This means that his experience with hemodialysis was based on seeing outpatients, not hospital ICU patients. Hemodialysis is different from continuous dialysis, and is often used for different reasons. Part of his unfamiliarity with the treatment was likely one of the reasons he didn't want to initiate CRRT. And yet, given the situation, why wouldn't the subbing nephrologist defer to someone with clear knowledge and experience? Looking back, Crystal thinks that it could have been a bit of medical chauvinism as well. "I think some physicians— and I don't know if this was the case with him, I didn't know this nephrologist, I'd never met him, and I usually do know them, and they know which nurses are knowledgeable about this—but I think some are like, 'Who are *you* to tell me how to run my practice?'"

Stalled by a doctor's firm and authoritative refusal, it's easiest to drop the issue. Many nurses would, Crystal knows. No matter how dedicated a nurse is to patient care, there are some issues that seem impossible to confront. But Crystal also knows she is right. Her reputation for being outspoken is something she's proud of. She isn't ready to give up fighting for her patient. "It's my personal responsibility. If I don't speak up and say something, it may mean the patient doesn't get the treatment they need. If I don't speak up and say something about the treatment they need, it may mean the patient's demise."

Crystal believes part of the difficulty in training nurses to speak up is the result of larger social issues. "It hasn't always been a culture where the nurses can do that. Historically, it's been almost a subservient type of profession where you follow orders. Yours is not to question; yours is just to carry out orders. We have to break that culture and that way of thinking. It's not the easiest thing, because it's also part of a personal culture. As women, we're taught not to question men, not to question authority, or we're taught not to question people older than us. So these are a part of the barrier that needs to be broken down."

Crystal has some experience with barriers. "As a kid, I was always the person to ask why we did certain things. I grew up Southern Baptist in Stone Mountain, Georgia. Part of our religion is to not ask 'Why?' It's to just have faith. But I always asked why." Ten-year-old Crystal asked why God would only allow Baptists into heaven, which would place everyone else, after death, squarely in hell. "I just couldn't understand why the loving God that I believed in would allow other religious people who believed in God, not necessarily Christ, to go to hell." The answer she usually got was some version of "Just because," and that rankled. Twenty-five years later, that answer, though given in a different context, still provokes Crystal. "I don't think in the healthcare field we should settle for the status quo, or with the answer that 'this is what we have always done and that's why we do it.' If you can't answer why we do it, then you need to look into it and find out why we do it."

"Crystal kept going back to her research and didn't back down," recalls Caryl, another ICU nurse who walked in on the tail end of the conversation between Crystal and Dr. Eff. The deadlock was simple: the attending nephrologist wanted to wait until the patient didn't have any kidney function left before considering a change in the current treatment, and Crystal wanted to start the treatment immediately. With improved dialysis intervention methods, the frequency of death due to uremia, hyperkalemia, and other kinds of electrolyte and metabolic imbalances has decreased. CRRT extracts the obstructive myoglobin molecules from the blood, which alleviates additional strain on already overtaxed kidneys: "If you remove the Jell-O and just filter water, eventually the water will help flush through the remaining Jell-O and begin to filter the water more rapidly," Crystal explains.

Mrs. Rhabdo cries while Crystal explains that the attending nephrologist refused to order the treatment. She has sat beside her husband all afternoon, and she knows without being told that he is getting worse. After Dr. Eff leaves without speaking to anyone else, Crystal gives the wife a hug and reassures her, "We're not done yet. Give us some time. This isn't over."

• • •

Critically ill patients often cannot speak for themselves, nor can family members always successfully negotiate layers of medical jargon and emotional overload. Doctors juggle heavy caseloads and often have little time to spare for second-guessing, diplomacy, or more than a cursory bedside nod. Nurses spend twelve-hour shifts several days a week with their patients, and their understanding of a patient's needs must be respected, too. Crystal explains that "a large part of nursing is being a patient advocate. Part of our profession, part of what nurses do, is being a voice for patients and their families. We're with patients 24/7, and the doctors are getting a snapshot view of the patient when they do their rounds. They normally have eighty patients or so, and it's up to us to convey that information to the doctors."

Being educated and knowing the literature creates a kind of respect. If the respect level is higher, people—doctors—will listen to nurses. Chief trauma resident Dr. Enn has worked with most of these nurses for "seventy-five percent of the last five years," and she attests to their high level of skill and knowledge. "They really pay attention to what's going on," she says. "They're always on top of things. I trust them emphatically."

The stand-in nephrologist, Dr. Eff, is neither familiar with nor trusting of the Trauma/ICU nurses at this facility. He is, thanks to Crystal, getting a whiplash-quick orientation. Earlier in the day, Crystal had asked him to phone Dr. Gee, to create what is called a "mutual purpose" for the patient's care, a request Dr. Eff ignored. Running high on emotion as well as the certainty that she is right, Crystal phones the chief primary care resident. Dr. Gee backs her up again, "You tell them that they will start it or we will find someone who will." This sounds a lot like an ultimatum, and Crystal's mind races for a diplomatic way to phrase the order as she dials Dr. Eff's pager number.

When Dr. Eff calls back, Crystal relays the message. "The primary team really wants CRRT started for this patient. That's why they consulted you, and they'd like you to reconsider."

When Crystal was eight years old, her mother got a job working as a crime scene investigator for the DeKalb County Police Department—"before it was cool, before *CSI* and all those other shows." Crystal, now thirty-five, isn't sure whether her mother's unusual profession influenced her own highly developed drive for clarity and accountability. "*Maybe*. Maybe that is true," she says, carefully weighing her words. "I've never thought about it that way. Could be."

And how much of what happened to her father when she was young influenced Crystal's chosen path? Her thirty-year-old father had a cerebral hemorrhage and was in the hospital for a year. Hospital policies were different then, and they tried to shield children from exposure to illness and injury. That kind of subterfuge must have been frustrating for an inquisitive child, the same child who would grow up and become committed to fostering clear and open dialogue.

Her mother had two children and a seriously debilitated husband to look after. And she never questioned that responsibility, Crystal remembers: "She just did what had to be done." Crystal's father also taught her important lessons in facing tough challenges. The doctors said he would never walk, talk, or see again. "I remember sitting down with him and his speech books. He had to learn everything all over again. How to walk, talk, how to process everything." With the exception of a vision problem, he made a complete recovery.

Shannon, one of Crystal's co-workers, confesses that she had a pretty hard time with Crystal's head-on, persistent style. "I thought she was just aggressive, condescending, and overly ambitious. I walked into a meeting one day, and Crystal had all of this stuff she brought in about Crucial Conversations that seemed like a huge waste of time, and I thought, 'Oh, she's really done it now.'" But one day, Shannon saw Crystal comfort a new nurse who was distraught about a patient who had died. The way Crystal supported the nurse made Shannon rethink her assessment. It didn't happen overnight, but she admits that over time she began to see two things: Crystal was able to talk about problems without talking about people, and other nurses supported Crystal because her methods work. Another ICU nurse, Caryl, adds, "When Crystal steps in, people don't get offended because they know she's stepping in to help. She's about empowering instead of blaming." Penny, who has worked with Crystal for six years, says that Crystal used to come off as more aggressive, but that when she softened her approach, a lot more nurses started to listen. But she also believes Crystal had to be aggressive at first, in order to get people to start looking at the problem. Shannon, the co-worker who admits to having been against Crystal's methods in the beginning, now says, "Crystal has given us all permission to speak out, and she has showed us how by example."

Nurses at this hospital are outspoken when they need to be, and they are encouraged to have open discussions and journal-sharing sessions, and to publish their stories in nursing journals and newsletters. Crystal wrote an account of Mr. Rhabdo's story for a Vital Smarts personal story contest, and won. After winning the contest, she attended a Crucial Conversations/AACN seminar in Washington, D.C. Obviously, Crystal has an innate sense of the importance of speaking out, but some of what she learned about softening her approach with co-workers came from what she learned at the seminar. She frequently uses Crucial Conversations training materials in staff meetings, and she recently submitted a proposal to bring Crucial Conversations training to Tampa. The issues raised by the Vital Smarts study and the Crucial Conversations training aid her work just as medical research helps her to successfully challenge a doctor's decision. The *Silence Kills* study is compelling, and the Vital Smarts books and methods back up what she's trying to make happen in the medical environment.

Crystal is generous in pointing out examples of how supportive and empowering the hospital is of their nursing staff. Even so, she says sometimes she feels there are negative consequences for being vocal: "Recently I didn't get a promotion, even though I was *probably* the most qualified person for the position. I was given the impression that I might not be the right fit, that they wanted someone who wouldn't be so likely to speak up as much as I do. You know, someone who doesn't speak up, who doesn't cause 'problems' in the way that I do. They didn't really say that. But it was made clear to me that they chose someone who never encountered 'problems.'"

Though Crystal targets communication problems with considerable zeal and idealism, she will also tell you accepting fallibility is a crucial factor in clear and effective interaction. "We're not always going to have perfect days, make the right decision, or even say the right thing," she says. "The most important thing is that we correct or make the situation right in the end. Most of the time, that means we have to admit we are not perfect, and then talk about what happened." Sometimes our filters get clogged, and emotions release in a flood. Sometimes crucial conversations don't work. But more importantly, sometimes they do.

Dr. Fellow and the attending nephrology physician are back in the Trauma/ICU. They finish writing the orders for CRRT treatment without speaking to Crystal. Her shift is nearly done. "Thank you for coming back. I know you didn't want to do this." The two doctors ignore her thanks. Crystal shrugs it off. This is what she calls a "silence instead of violence" kind of response.

Within twenty-four hours after the treatment begins, Mr. Rhabdo starts to improve. He'll spend several more weeks in the Trauma/ICU, but he and Mrs. Rhabdo will celebrate Christmas and welcome the New Year on another floor of the hospital, not in Intensive Care. They are profuse in expressing their gratitude for Crystal's intervention. "The wife, being a nurse, understood that it's not always easy to speak up, and that there are these kinds of conflicts. She doesn't feel like he would have gotten the care if I hadn't spoken up," Crystal says. When Crystal's essay about Mr. Rhabdo's case comes out in Vital Smarts a few months later, she goes up to his floor and gives them a copy. It is a celebration of much more than winning a writing contest.

Since the publication of her essay on the Vital Smarts Web site and after Crystal attended the conference in D.C., Crystal's peers have started coming to her with questions like, "I need to have this conversation, but how do you think I should approach so-and-so?" or "My babysitter isn't doing what I think she should, so how can I correct her without hurting her feelings?" or "Help! I need to have a Crucial Conversation." It's routine for the nurses in this unit to question each other or give advice, especially from more- to less-experienced nurses. They take pride in their commitment to patient safety and optimal outcomes, and learning Crucial Conversation skills raises the standard of care, which, every ICU nurse will tell you, is the bottom line. The nurses take pride in their ability to communicate more "fluidly," as Crystal describes it. "We can hold each other accountable. We can be responsible for change."

Jill Drumm is a poet and writer living in Fort Myers, Florida. She received her MFA in Creative Writing from Florida International University (Miami) and teaches writing at Florida Gulf Coast University. Her work has appeared or is forthcoming in *TriQuarterly*, *Margie Review*, *RUNES: A Review of Poetry*, *Florida English*, and *Gulf Stream*.

About the Editor

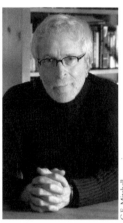

LEE GUTKIND's most recent book, *Almost Human: Making Robots Think,* details his experiences at the Robotics Institute at Carnegie-Mellon University. His immersion into the motorcycle subculture (*Bike Fever*), the organ transplant milieu (*Many Sleepless Nights*), and other previously un-mined worlds has led to nine books and many awards for his literary achievements. He is a professor of English at the University of Pittsburgh and founder and editor of the literary journal *Creative Nonfiction*.